this is

post

partum

this is post

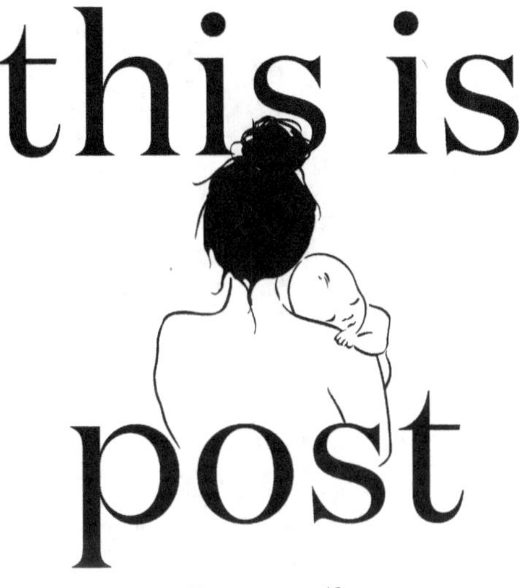

Free yourself
from the perfect mother conspiracy

partum

Tilda Timmers

This edition was published by The Dreamwork Collective
The Dreamwork Collective LLC, Dubai, United Arab Emirates
thedreamworkcollective.com

Printed and bound in the United Arab Emirates
Cover Design: Heike Schüssler

Copyright © Tilda Timmers, 2020

ISBN 9789948354420
Approved by National Media Council
Dubai, United Arab Emirates
MC-02-01-2914492

This book is not intended as a substitute for the medical or mental health advice of professionals. The reader should regularly consult a physician and/or mental health professional in matters relating to their health and wellbeing, particularly with respect to any symptoms that may require diagnosis or medical attention.

To all the moms out there who
struggle and feel like a failure:
I see you. I feel you.
You are good enough!

Table of Contents

Introduction

This is my life . . .
My story . . . my book.
I will no longer let anyone else write it
Nor will I apologize
For the edits I make

Who is this book for?

- Have you just had a baby and feel ashamed that you're not feeling as blissful as you thought you would be? Do you feel afraid and alone?
- Do you feel like no one understands you, or that people think you're not a good mother?
- Do you cry with pain during breastfeeding but grit your teeth because of your mother-in-law's comments?
- Do you scroll through endless Happy Mommy Instagram accounts, wondering what the hell is wrong with you?

If you answered yes to any of these questions, please read this book. You're not alone. Whether or not your symptoms fit a specific diagnosis or label that society has come up with, the bottom line is this: You don't feel your best right now, and you want to feel better. Being a mom is hard. For every woman. Even the ones who look like they've got it totally sorted. (Especially those ones?) My book will help you through this difficult period and encourage you to embrace the inevitable joys and tears.

After giving birth to my oldest daughter, Livia, I was as far from that image of a proud, radiant new mom on cloud nine as it is possible to be. I felt like my throat was being squeezed and I couldn't get any air—like I was slowly drowning. It was as if someone had thrown a huge, dark blanket over me. When I looked at my baby, I was both madly in love with her and filled with terror. *What if something happens to her?* The anxiety was oppressive and I became more insecure every day. I didn't know what to do about how I felt and, bit by bit, I lost myself. Eventually I was diagnosed with postpartum depression (PPD). Wanting to be the perfect mother had paralyzed me. And what *is* a perfect mother anyway? If you're not (as we say in Dutch) on a pink cloud after giving birth, but on a stifling grey one, you'll want to do everything in your power to change how you feel. PPD can feel suffocating, absolutely unbearable. What makes it worse is that it's so hard to talk about. That's understandable, because whether you're facing postpartum depression or simply finding motherhood difficult, admitting that to yourself and others is not easy. It requires self-awareness and a huge dose of courage because unfortunately, society still has very judgmental attitudes about motherhood and how things should be done. A friend who wouldn't dream of telling you how to dress is suddenly telling you what to do with your breasts.

But speaking out is vital. You don't have to go through this alone!

I wrote this book for two types of mothers: those with PPD and those who don't have it but still occasionally struggle with motherhood and all that it involves. PPD is incredibly common, but at the same time, you don't have to be diagnosed with it to feel that motherhood can be rough, even a bit hellish sometimes. But if you do have postpartum depression or you think you have it, don't rely on this book alone; please also get professional help as soon as possible.

In this book you'll find ideas to make your life easier after childbirth. Each chapter is divided into bite-size subtopics, so you can quickly scan what's relevant to you at that particular moment. I've tried and tested all the tips and tricks, and my clients have found them useful, too. I discuss the benefits of mindfulness and how this can help you relate to your negative feelings in a very different way. I also give you my take on the breast versus bottle debate, how sharing your feelings is vital, and how exercise can help you recover from depression. Of course, this is all just advice, nothing prescriptive, and as a mother you should always consider all the options and do what suits you best.

Note: For ease of writing I use 'he' or 'she' interchangeably, but the words cover both male and female babies and adults. And even though I often refer to partners as men, of course I also mean female partners.

Despite how horrible I felt during my postpartum depression, the experience helped me find my true purpose. The support I received during my recovery made it clear to me that I wanted to help others in the same way I had been helped. A nurse made a very sweet comment when several of my friends came over, the week after the delivery. My friends had been telling me about their problems and issues, and my nurse said, 'Wow, Tilda. You give such amazing advice to your friends. You should do something with that.' The comment stuck with me, and thanks to it, after months of crying, worrying, and little sleep, I trained as a therapist so I could put all my experiences and new knowledge into helping other mothers. I truly hope this book helps you get that much needed air and space for yourself again, and I thank you for coming on this journey with me.

The Perfect Mother Conspiracy

When you first become a mother, you're likely to put a great deal of pressure on yourself to be a very 'good' mother. You feel like you want to be the best version of motherhood there could possibly be. Problem is, there's no such thing as a perfect mother. It simply doesn't exist. In the Netherlands, we have a saying: 'Perfect mothers aren't real. And real mothers aren't perfect.'

When you look around—in the local park, within your friendship group, on social media—you might be forgiven for thinking that all the mothers you see are perfect. That they don't struggle with motherhood or that they always feel confident and competent. Nothing could be further from the truth. I can't stress that enough. What you see on social media are only the most photogenic aspects of their lives. Maybe they're struggling, maybe they just had a fight with their partner, maybe their mothers were criticizing their parenting skills all morning, maybe they're wondering why *you* look so calm and peaceful. But they don't put that on social media, do they? They only show you the so-called perfect version: that smiling little baby boy next to a blooming houseplant. Or photos of a week's worth of colourful organic vegan meals. I mean, who *does* that? Ain't nobody got time for that! Especially not with a newborn. I was happy if I remembered to order my Thai food early enough so I didn't have to eat at midnight.

It feels almost like there's a Perfect Mother Conspiracy. Even seemingly innocent magazine articles—"Snap back into shape in six weeks"—perpetuate the myth of this feminine-mother ideal, that there's only one way of feeling good, looking good, being 'good'. What rubbish! I remember wanting to be that perfect mom. I didn't want to admit to myself or anyone else that I felt like a failure 99 percent of the time. I watched all the Insta-perfect celebrity moms and thought, *I can never live up to that. I must be a terrible mother.*

For starters, I didn't fit into my skinny jeans after six weeks. Let's be totally frank: My youngest child is now two years old, and if I try my very best and suck in my tummy like crazy and lie down, I *might* fit into that old pair of jeans. If I so much as sit up or breathe, they'll pop open. But really, who cares? Perhaps that's been one of my biggest and most transformative journeys as a mother. There was a time when things like that would have really bothered me. Now, after much work on myself (which I'll share with you in this book), I can truly say, hand on heart, that I value and love myself in a way I never did before. The main message I have for you in this book is to be truly kind to yourself and lower the bar as much as possible. In doing so, you'll 'achieve' way more than you would if you aimed for perfection, and you'll also give yourself the space to work out what your values are, what matters to you, which won't necessarily be the values society imposes on us. For example, by allowing myself to stop caring about having an immaculately clean house, I gave myself more time to realise that housekeeping isn't one of my core values, but working and connecting with other moms really is.

My answer to the Perfect Mother Conspiracy is this: Let's normalise not feeling on cloud nine after childbirth. New parenthood is not always easy, so let's please be open about all the stuff nobody talks about. It's completely fine to find parenthood hellish at times. It doesn't mean you're a bad parent, and it doesn't mean you don't adore your child. I want to free you from feeling that you're not good enough and to make you feel confident as a new parent. I want you to feel calmer, knowing that this is just a phase and you won't feel like this forever. You'll get through this first stage as a new parent: this crazy, chaotic, sleep-deprived phase that sometimes makes you want to scream.

Some mothers reading this book will be struggling with occasional anxiety, whereas other moms will have (or suspect) a postpartum depression diagnosis. Whether it is the former or the latter or anything in between, this book is for you, dear mother.

It doesn't matter how you label your experience (I prefer no labels at all, honestly); what matters is healing yourself, being kind to yourself, and knowing that you *will* get through this. Step by step, one day at a time.

Let this book be a beacon of hope in challenging times. May this book support you and bring you the self-esteem you long for and so immensely deserve. I'm here for you. When you're up breastfeeding in the middle of the night and feeling lonely, I'm your ally.

This. Is. Post. Partum. Nothing more, nothing less. Welcome, and enjoy the ride!

CHAPTER 1

Two New Mothers, Two Different Realities

Don't be ashamed of your story
It will inspire others

My story

It's 2014. I have a newborn baby girl, Livia, and I don't feel like myself at all. Our friends obviously want to come over and meet her right away. I don't want to see any of them; I just want to be left alone. My parents, my parents-in-law, and some of my best friends come by. Because of the stitches down under, I can barely sit, stand, or walk. This leaves me with few options. I feel exhausted, a walking zombie. I can barely talk. I just want to sleep. I pretend I'm feeling fine and that I have my act together. But I don't. Inside I'm terrified. I ask myself on a daily basis, *How do other mothers do this, this thing called motherhood?*

I just don't feel like seeing anyone. In the evenings, I cry for hours. I cannot deal with anything or anyone. No music, no television, and good luck anyone who so much as dares watch the news while I'm in the same room.

It was obvious that I was really struggling. At the end of the first week, I think I'd shed more tears than I'd ever shed before. I was completely drained. I clung to a nurse and asked, 'Is this normal? I think I'm having postpartum depression.' She looked at me and replied that I was just very disrupted by the hormones and lack of sleep. I should sleep with earplugs that night and take a sleeping pill and my husband would do the night feeds. 'Then you'll feel a lot better tomorrow.' She was right; I did feel a little better the next morning. But not the days after. Nor the weeks and months after that, either.

I slipped further and further into depression. I had many depressive thoughts, fluctuating between *I should never have become a mother* to *I want to die.* I worried about everything: whether I was a good mother and if I was the only woman on Earth who wasn't capable of being a good mother. When my daughter slept at night, I lay awake, worrying. When someone unexpectedly swung by to say hi and admire Liv, I freaked out. And when I left Liv at home, even if just to buy some groceries, I checked my phone every two minutes to make sure there hadn't been a disaster. I stopped meeting up with friends. My self-deprecation and sense of humour disappeared. Where had I gone?

I became more and more silent, my thoughts progressively darker. When I walked over a bridge with my baby in the pram, I thought, *If I let go of her now, the pram will speed down the bridge and she'll be dead.* And when I walked past the stairs of our apartment complex, I thought, *If I overturn the pram, she'll be dead.* I felt so ashamed of those thoughts, but I couldn't block them out. I thought I'd never be able to forgive myself for thinking such terrible things.

One night I realized that I had to voice some of this to my husband. As lightly as possible, I said, 'Sometimes I think our daughter deserves a better mother than me.' He looked at me, stunned, eyes widening, and said, 'Well, honey, you can't say that to me! I'm really shocked when you say stuff like this. Of course you're a great mother.' I was so startled by his shocked face that I thought, *Okay, I don't want him to worry about me. He'll start to think I'm crazy. I'll keep it to myself. It'll be fine.*

What made the first months of motherhood extra hard for me was that my grandmother passed away when I was 22 weeks pregnant. She was a key figure in my life, and when she suddenly passed away, my world was turned upside down. This woman, who had been a role model to me, a huge source of inspiration, would never meet my daughter, and I would have to go through this special time in my life without her.

Grandma taught me how to walk in heels by the age of seven. My very first pair of heels were hers. Her backyard became my runway. As well as wearing high heels, she also loved to curl her hair, put on lipstick, and spray herself lavishly with nice cologne. Invariably, before we went grocery shopping, she made sure her lipstick was immaculate. I think my love for lip gloss was born then. Grandma followed fashion trends religiously. Every time I came into her house in a nice dress, she'd say, 'Yes, that colour is completely in style again.' She couldn't reach her toes anymore so, from a very young age, I painted her toenails for her, something I did with a lot of love. She was very proud of her well-groomed toes. When someone complimented her on her nails, she'd say proudly, 'My granddaughter did a great job.'

Her death was, as I said, very unexpected. She died of pneumonia within a day. While I was watching over her next to her hospital bed, I kept wondering how this could be happening. My dearest, dearest grandmother was dying and there was nothing I could do. I stroked her wrinkled hands and whispered in her ear that it was okay. 'You may go, my love, you've given us so much. Thanks to you, I'm the person I have become. You were a great grandmother.' My husband sent me home late at night, and he took over from me. She passed away at 1 a.m. Two hours later, Nelson Mandela passed away as well. She could not have wished for better company during her crossing.

The week after her passing, I was in a daze. I went to the funeral centre every day to sit next to her, talk to her. We burned scented candles and listened to music, because Grandma loved music so much. Again and again, I touched her hands. Now they were freezing cold, just like her face. I was in shock. The cremation was hell. When we finally had to leave the coffin, I cuddled it with both arms, hysterically crying. When I think back to it now, I still get goose bumps all over my body.

Of course, I wondered whether this enormous loss would affect my mental health after giving birth. I discussed my concern during my many visits to the gynaecologist. But because everyone kept saying that they didn't know, or that it would be okay, or that we would see when the time came, I left it.

Even without a death in the family, some new mothers might experience feelings of grief, perhaps because they don't have a good relationship with their own mother. Becoming a mother can then be extra complicated. My relationship with my mother wasn't great when I was growing up. My grandmother was my safe haven. I'd go to her house often to find shelter and feel loved and accepted. My gran and I were so close and we could understand each other without saying a word. She was a wonderful role model for me, for the kind of mother I wanted to be for my children. Her absence when Livia was born was heart-breaking. Honestly, it still is very painful. I miss her so much.

Two weeks after Livia's birth, I decided to call my former psychologist, the one who worked with me during the grieving process for my grandmother. She had helped me a great deal and I felt a very strong connection with her. At the start of my therapy sessions I didn't have the courage to tell her immediately about the dark thoughts I was having about Liv. I felt so ashamed. Fortunately, she asked me a lot of thorough questions and after five sessions, I finally plucked up the courage to tell her what was really going on in my head. She replied, 'Tilda, like many other mothers, you're suffering from intrusions. These are compulsive thoughts that the vast majority of mankind also have. Most people let go of the thoughts just as easily as they come up. You, however, are viewing them with a magnifying glass. As a result, they get bigger and worse in your head.' Then she said, 'You have postpartum depression.'

Aha! This was a huge eye-opener for me. *Intrusions.* I wanted to know more, but my husband had banned me from googling anything at that time, because I became obsessed about whatever I read on the internet. My therapist also recommended avoiding the internet, because I was driving myself crazy googling *everything.* Even whether penguins had knees! So she printed an article about intrusions from *Psychologies Magazine* and I read it repeatedly until the edges of the paper were frayed and curled. It helped me stop being so afraid of the intrusions.

There are some misconceptions about PPD: People have images of a mother not loving her baby or neglecting her child. I didn't hide my child in a cardboard box, nor did I pretend she didn't exist. Instead, I was overly anxious and panicky that something bad would happen to her, which made me unable to see the joy in living. I had intrusive thoughts about my baby, myself, and Tim. I was worried out of my mind that, thanks to me, something awful would happen to Liv. I didn't eat, I didn't sleep, and I didn't talk about any of my negative thoughts or feelings because I felt so guilty and ashamed of them. The control freak in me worked overtime, and on the inside I slowly became a staggeringly uncertain version of myself.

After eight months I noticed that my depression was beginning to ease. I remembered the nurse's comment, and I started thinking about what I really wanted to do with my life. In retrospect, the depression turned out to be a way of resetting my brain. Gradually I noticed that there was room in my head to think about the future. I wanted nothing more than to help other mothers, so I trained as a therapist and started my practice for other mothers who feel like they can't breathe, who feel suffocated by everything that's going on in their lives, who need help and guidance through a difficult time. My coaching company is called Frou Frou, which comes from the memories I have of my grandmother. She was my confidante, my life coach. While enjoying a pot of tea and her favourite cookies (Frou Frous), I could tell her about anything and everything. I want my clients to feel as safe and secure with me as I felt with my grandmother.

Sophie's Story

Sophie, one of my clients, said, 'I don't know where to turn to with my negative thoughts about being a mom. I feel completely unable to do this thing called motherhood and I feel like I'm failing on a daily basis.' Sophie felt very ashamed about not enjoying being a mother. Because she was the first one in her group of friends to have a child, she didn't have any mom friends to talk to, and her normal friends didn't get what she was talking about. They'd say, 'Why aren't you coming to lunch with us? Just bring the baby.' But Sophie was afraid her baby wouldn't fall asleep and would cry. Plus, she didn't want her baby to fall out of her routine. So she stayed inside and felt lonelier every day.

Sophie is far from alone. It's extremely common for new mothers to not feel good in the first months. Not all these women have PPD; some simply feel overwhelmed. Completely understandable, if you ask me. Becoming a mother is intense. You suddenly have an entire new role that no one has prepared you for, a role filled with new responsibilities. It can feel like sitting exams you haven't studied for. If you were starting a new job, there would likely be a handover period, or there would be people in the office you could question and have a chat with. But many mothers spend large portions of their days alone. Over and over again, day in and day out. That's hard, so of course sometimes you feel like you can't do it.

Sophie came to me to talk about her negative thoughts and the way she tormented herself with worry, especially at night. She felt at ease with me and dared to share her deepest and darkest thoughts. After six sessions, she felt much better and more confident as a mother. She still emails me about how she's doing, and I couldn't be prouder of her. In the following chapters I go into detail about some of the ideas I shared with Sophie and many other mothers who came to my practice.

What Sophie had in common with a lot of new moms is that she worried she wasn't good enough. Nobody likes the feeling of not being good enough. The feeling eats away at you and before you know it, you start confusing your thoughts with facts and you actually come to believe that you *aren't* good enough.

For Sophie, what made her negative thoughts worse was the way she was always comparing herself to other mothers. Maybe you're the same: You see all the other moms in your mommy group thriving. Maybe you see your friends 'doing' motherhood seemingly effortlessly. And let's not forget about the so-called perfect Insta-moms with their flawless makeup, stylish outfits, and smiling babies. We end up thinking, *How come I'm struggling so much and they're not? How come I can't even get out of bed today?* These comparisons make everything worse, so one of the first things I recommend to my clients is this: Stop comparing yourself to others! I'll give you tips on how to break out of this habit later, but for now, just remember that the grass is always greener because it is most likely fake.

Sophie and I, in our different ways, struggled just like you're struggling right now. I remember the feeling of incompetence so vividly; it's a terrible feeling. But remember, your success as a mother doesn't depend on your subjective thoughts about yourself as a mother. Are you talking yourself down a lot? If you set the bar too high, you'll set yourself up for failure, so be gentle with yourself. You're doing the best you can. I hope you can find some comfort in that thought. Being a mother can be brutal sometimes, but it can also be the best thing that will ever happen to you. The fact that you don't feel that way right now doesn't mean you will never feel it. Trust the process. It will all come your way eventually.

When you decided you wanted to have a child, you probably had big dreams and deep thoughts about motherhood, hopes and dreams for your baby, and for yourself as a mother but also as a couple (if you have a partner). Subconsciously, you already set the bar very high. Most of the women who come to my practice did that without even realizing it. They set the bar insanely high. It would be impossible for *anyone* to meet the standards they set for themselves, and naturally they felt a complete sense of failure on a daily basis. They constantly felt like they weren't good enough.

Let me emphasise this: All new parents feel unsure. Those first nights when you're home alone with your inconsolable baby are tough. Often mothers tell me, 'I was just sitting there, looking at my partner like, what the hell is happening? Why can't I calm my own baby? Why won't she stop crying?' They feel incapable and that's when the seeds of insecurity start to sprout. You don't want that to happen, of course, but it often does. It's common and normal, and you mostly don't even realize it's happening.

After a while, the feeling of not being capable of being a good mother can start to fester. It spreads through your brain, and before you know it, anything and everything that goes wrong on any given day is your fault. The baby doesn't sleep during the day: *Must be my fault.* The little one refuses to drink: *Must be because I'm not a good mom.* What most new mothers don't realize is that babies do their own thing 24/7. They're not robots, so they won't act or react the same way every day. When your baby doesn't feed well or doesn't sleep a lot, it isn't your fault. Maybe he just wants to be close to you, or maybe he has stomach cramps and drinking makes it worse. You never know for sure, because unfortunately, babies can't yet talk. Biggest bummer ever, if you ask me. So, if they can only communicate through crying, obviously they have to cry a lot. What else can they do? If you're feeling like a failure, please listen to me when I say that you're not. Like Sophie, you're just struggling to adjust to your new role.

Talking openly about these struggles is very difficult for most of us because of the pressure and expectation for new parents to be completely over the moon at all times. #blessed. We feel ashamed and guilty that we don't enjoy motherhood some or even most of the time. We don't want people to see us as a bad mother or to think that we're a failure. These are very real fears, and they keep us from opening up. But once you do talk about your struggles and fears, you'll hear similar stories from friends, relatives, or colleagues who know someone who was in the same boat. Mothers who struggled in the past will recognize their own stories in what you're saying. Knowing that you're not alone is very important on your road to recovery.

Make no mistake, not feeling like you're on cloud nine after giving birth is common. That first period after delivery is intense and sometimes very hard. Take your distress seriously and be as kind to yourself as possible. Don't judge yourself for your feelings but do lower the bar and be realistic. You don't have to be the perfect parent, because that's not even possible. All you have to be is a good parent for your baby, and you already are.

Realizing Things Aren't Quite Right

Post natal depression
is an illness
Not a reflection of you
as a mother or as a woman

My 35-year-old client Marianne was completely desperate because she wasn't sleeping. Her baby turned out to be one of those nonstop crying babies. Sometimes she had thoughts such as, *If I put a pillow over her head now, it's all over.* Of course, she was very upset by those thoughts, and they would be swiftly followed by: *I'm a bad mother.* Like many mothers who suffer from PPD, Marianne was experiencing intrusive thoughts. She also told me she'd been getting so absentminded that she even once forgot to fasten her baby's car seat belt. She didn't tell anyone about that because she felt too guilty. And so she got progressively more lonely.

Right after giving birth, a lot of new mothers suffer from crying episodes, irritability, nervousness, and sleep problems. This period is also called the baby blues, and according to the National Institute of Mental Health[1], up to 80 percent of new mothers experience it. The baby blues are particularly prevalent from the third day until about the tenth day after delivery, but this varies. For some women, the symptoms start a few weeks after giving birth or even much later, when they go back to work. The symptoms usually pass after a couple of weeks.

The baby blues become problematic when the depressive mood persists. Headaches, irritability, loss of appetite, crying, and poor sleep should set off your alarm bells. Most women I see in my practice notice quite quickly that things aren't right. They tend to contact me when their babies are anything between two and twenty weeks old. Please, please, please, if you're suffering from ongoing symptoms like these, seek help as soon as possible. The sooner you ask for help or treatment, the better. Trust your gut on this; you don't have to wait months to get the help you need right now.

Causes of PPD

The risk of a woman suffering from depression triples in the first month after delivery, compared with childless women of the same age. Fluctuating hormones make mothers more vulnerable to depression, but difficult psychosocial conditions also increase susceptibility. Such conditions might be one of the following:

- You have a bad relationship with your parents.
- You have lost your mother or a key figure in your life.
- Your parents or close family live far away.
- You want to keep everything under control.
- You have very high expectations of yourself and of life in general.
- You have an argument with people in your social circle.
- You have problems at work.
- You have financial difficulties or debts.
- You are in a toxic relationship and/or have experienced domestic violence.
- You have had mental health issues in the past.

The recent increase in the prevalence of PPD is likely, in part, to be related to the increase in psychosocial problems in society. It takes a village to raise a child, but nowadays we don't have that village. In the past, most mothers could lean on their own mother, who was often at home. These days, grandmothers often have their own career, or are divorced, or live far away, or sometimes live with a new partner and stepchildren. In some cases, the grandmothers themselves have started a new family or are very busy with their own lives. For any number of reasons, they're less available to help their daughter and new grandchild. The new mothers are therefore more dependent on themselves.

And then there's the Perfect Mother Conspiracy. There's judgment regarding whether or not we choose to nurse, whether we've 'succeeded' in getting our baby to sleep through the night, and what kind of routine we've perfected. And don't get me started on the pressure to lose the dreaded baby weight. Mother and baby groups can be immensely helpful, and at their best, lifelong friendships can be formed, but they can also leave us feeling inadequate, believing that everyone else is doing better than we are.

Your relationship with your parents

Sometimes, the growing distance to their own parents creates a difficult environment for new mothers. A young mother needs a lot of support. During the post-childbirth period, the search for a reference figure automatically starts: What is motherhood? What makes a woman a good mother? New mothers look back on their own childhood and sometimes relive traumatic childhood experiences. Psychoanalysts refer to this phenomenon as ghosts in the nursery. This certainly happened to me: I had a rather complicated relationship with my mother and a lot of difficult memories came up after I gave birth to my first child. My postpartum therapist helped me work through it, and I also did EMDR (Eye Movement Desensitization and Reprocessing—more on this later) to relieve my childhood traumas.

Mothers who were adopted or never knew their biological mother are also more affected by their new role. Sadness and other feelings relating to having never known their biological mother come to the surface intensely when they become mothers themselves. Similarly, women who no longer have a mother miss the enormous support that their mother could have given. They want to ask questions such as, 'Mom, how did you do this when I was little?', 'Did I cry a lot as a baby?', 'What was I like as a toddler?' I see this regularly with clients in my practice. The lack of their own mother is keenly felt.

Perfectionism

Postpartum depression is also more prevalent in mothers who have difficulty with role change. Any big role change and life upheaval takes some adjustment. But you might find it particularly difficult if you, like me, developed a lot of insecurities over the years and feel like you need to control everything, and you set the bar very high for yourself. This can get complicated, because a baby isn't something you can control. Having a baby is essentially a crash course in Letting Go.

Mothers often feel that everything has to go according to the book. Getting help is not a priority. This is a result of today's society where everything is (apparently) feasible: advertisements show perfect women, perfect relationships, and perfect families. And celebrities who post their blissful photos on Facebook and Instagram don't make it any easier. A vulnerable new mother sees these photos after childbirth and thinks, *Why don't I feel that way? Why isn't my stomach flat yet? Why can't I go outside for a nice walk with my baby?* It can push some mothers completely over the edge.

Many new mothers get overwhelmed by all the information they're meant to remember. A client once told me, 'I felt like I had to do a test, like in high school, and I always got a D.' I relate to that, and I see a lot of new moms in my practice who feel this way, too.

Signs of postpartum depression (if these symptoms last longer than 2 to 4 weeks, ask for help immediately)

- You're irritable.
- You can barely concentrate.
- You feel dejected.
- You sleep badly, even when your baby is asleep.
- You eat a lot or very little.
- You think about suicide or death.
- You have difficulty concentrating and making decisions.
- You lose interest in the world around you and no longer enjoy the things that used to give you pleasure.
- You feel that everything takes a lot of effort; you don't want to be asked for anything.
- You feel that you're outside of life.
- You have negative thoughts and feelings about motherhood.
- You cry a lot and often during the day.
- You're unreasonable and unkind to people in your immediate environment (family, friends, colleagues, etc.).
- You feel incredibly insecure and you put an enormous amount of pressure on yourself.
- You experience intrusive thoughts. For example: You vividly visualise throwing your baby down the stairs or choking your child.

Prenatal depression

I've now started treating pregnant women in my practice because expecting mothers came looking for help through my website and social media channels. Many women suffer from depression during their pregnancy. It's thought that lack of social support and presence of marital discord may increase the likelihood of this type of depression. Sadly, this is currently a neglected topic, with little research from which to draw guidelines and recommendations. Much more work needs to be done in this area.

However, many of the recommendations given to women with postpartum depression are also relevant if you're suffering from depression before you've had your baby. Seek help as soon as possible. I can't stress enough how important early intervention is. The sooner you get help, the better, although it's never too late to get help. Recovery is possible at any stage.

Intrusive thoughts: functional warnings

Everyone sometimes has thoughts that they really don't want to have. Maybe you recognize a situation like this: You bend over and admire your sister's new baby. You fall in love with your new niece immediately. Suddenly a thought flashes through your mind about how you could wrap your hands around this cute baby's throat and choke her. It's obviously the last thing in the world you want to do, but the scene in your mind is vivid and it horrifies you. Or you're at the train station. In the distance, the train is fast approaching. You see yourself walking to the edge of the platform and jumping off. You're thinking, *If I jump in front of the train now, the driver won't be able to stop in time.* The thought fills you with horror. Yet a little devil calls inside, 'Come on, do it!'

Thoughts about sex with your father-in-law are a more comically horrifying example of an intrusive thought. These types of thought are completely normal, even though they send chills running down your spine. Mothers who are naturally perfectionist are more likely to have these intrusions. Lack of sleep makes the tendency worse, and before you know it, these awful thoughts have taken over completely.

Nadine Rhoen, a child and family psychologist, explains the function of intrusions: 'An intrusion is a thought that just comes to mind and can be quite bizarre, even frightening. But having an intrusion is actually a way our brain protects us from inattention. Through the intrusive thought, you become aware of the serious consequences that the execution of such a thought would have, and it makes you realize that you should not do this. So it's actually a very good protection system made by the brain.'

Dutch psychologists Fred Sterk and Sjoerd Swaen[2] further confirm that intrusions are an evolutionary warning system designed to protect us from danger and inattention. We're all wired to be constantly on high alert for possible threats to our children. If you unexpectedly think of strangling a baby, you're being alerted to the vulnerability of small babies. When it comes to survival, our brain is not subtle; it is purely functional. These troubling thoughts stem from the mother's concern and her enormous sense of responsibility. Your brain wants to point out what could happen to your baby and that you have to stay alert. You absolutely do not have to be ashamed of having such thoughts.

Almost everyone has an intrusion on a daily basis. They get startled by it for a minute then continue with their day. If, on the other hand, you take the intrusions seriously, you might start obsessing about the thoughts and what is behind them. Then unimportant intrusions can become annoying and you can develop compulsions or fears. People think that pregnancy and birth are special, magical periods in a woman's life. If you have a lot of negative thoughts after you deliver your child, you might feel very sad and anxious, because you think you're 'meant' to be having a special, magical time. Intrusive thoughts can contribute to a feeling of depression because the thoughts can be so stressful to experience —a far cry from a special, magical time. What usually works best is to notice the thoughts, say to yourself gently, *Oh look, I'm having an intrusive thought'*, then direct your attention elsewhere. Easier said than done. I'll go into tips on how to do this in chapter 5. If you find that intrusions are stopping you doing certain things, seek help from a professional.

Getting professional help

I can't overemphasize the importance of getting help. It saved me. I had Cognitive Behaviour Therapy and I did a lot of mindfulness work. My therapist also gave me homework, which I gladly accepted. Anything to get out of the hell of PPD. I saw my therapist on a weekly basis at first, then when I started feeling better, every two weeks, then three, four, etc. Sometimes I called my therapist if I was feeling really low and couldn't wait until the next appointment, something I really appreciated being able to do. With good emotional and coaching support and practical help, recovery is absolutely possible.

If you feel well most of the time and only occasionally have milder symptoms of depression, you might prefer to talk to your partner or a good friend. The tips and advice in this book will still help you. But if you feel bad more often than not, or have intrusive thoughts that really upset you, or you're thinking about running away or killing yourself, it is crucial to get help. I strongly recommend you call your doctor or approach healthcare professionals immediately. Maybe you've read about a certain therapist who appealed to you. Please approach him or her and make an appointment as soon as possible. More details on this in the next chapter.

International research has shown that postpartum depression often goes undetected. This happens because most sufferers don't talk about it. These mothers feel guilty and ashamed, so they keep their thoughts and feelings to themselves. Because of this, other new mothers often don't know which signals are associated with this kind of depression. In this way, the cycle continues. Let's break the cycle!

CHAPTER 3

Breaking the Silence

A hopeless moment
Doesn't make you
A hopeless mother

It's very difficult to talk about the fact that you're not enjoying being a new mother. I remember feeling so ashamed of my thoughts, feeling so guilty about my negative feelings about motherhood. Many mothers feel the same and, unfortunately, many are silent about what's really going on inside their head. The taboo surrounding suffocating postpartum depression, or just not loving being a mother, continues. The saintly mother conspiracy tells us that women should love every moment of being a mother, that it's unnatural to not constantly feel full of love and nurturing affection. This makes me roll my eyes. A lot. Because no mother loves being a mother 24/7. And the women who do pretend that it's all fun and amazing? They're probably lying. Maybe even lying to themselves. In this chapter you'll learn why it's so important to share what's going on in your head.

Important: If you're experiencing the symptoms listed in chapter 2, please go straight to the section on getting professional help (page 45). Yes, talking to friends and family can help, and these people can play a big role in your recovery, but it is essential you get professional help, too.

Don't struggle alone

It takes courage to share your true feelings with others. I had such intense thoughts but kept trying to suppress them. Ever further and ever deeper, I pushed my 'crazy' thoughts back. I'd be unloading my dishwasher, and whenever my hands touched a knife, I'd see how I could stab my baby to death. It was the most gruesome and horrible thought I'd ever had. But I had it. Every day. The dishwasher didn't unload itself, and so I had to live with the intrusive thoughts. They were much too scary for me to handle.

My husband is a trauma surgeon, and when I was in the middle of my postpartum depression, I regularly cursed his long workdays. I was alone with our baby all day. I did the full shift, every day and most nights. It was tough. So tough that I started to blame him more and more. Of course, I knew in advance what I was getting into when I married him, and it's not like he had a choice about his working hours. But if you're a new mother who's feeling really dreadful, you're not always open to reason. Sometimes, you just want someone to take over. I stayed silent as my depression intensified and my anger toward my husband grew and grew. I didn't share my true thoughts and feelings with anyone and so they snowballed, up until the moment where I thought, *I don't want to live like this anymore. I can't do this anymore. I don't want this for me or my family.*

I'd tried to tell my husband how bad I felt, but because I'd been vague and expressed myself in a clumsy way, he'd just been very shocked. I remember making a conscious decision to stop sharing my crazy thoughts with him. I didn't want to do that to him, to drag him along with me in my grief. No, I wasn't going to do that. I'd do it alone, by myself; just keep going, head up, shoulders back, that was the way.

Except it wasn't. Not at all. After almost ten weeks, I was at the bottom of the very deepest pit I had ever been in. Then my best friend called. It seems that she knows me better than I know myself, because she'd known for a long time that I'd completely lost myself. She told me that I was acting strangely, saying things that I'd never normally say, and was sometimes downright unkind. 'What's going on, Til?' she asked. I broke down. I broke into a thousand pieces. On the phone, all I could do was cry, scream, and rage. I didn't tell her everything, nowhere close, but finally I'd started to share my true feelings. I told her I was afraid I might hurt my child. Obviously, she asked what I meant, but I said I couldn't tell her, that it was too bad. She then said that I had to promise her I'd speak to my therapist. I promised, and eventually I did tell my therapist everything.

Thanks to that conversation with my best friend, the negative cycle was broken and I was released from my homemade armour. Thanks to her, I found the courage to be completely honest during therapy sessions and also, later, with my husband. I'm so grateful for that conversation and will remain so until my dying day. Without it, I might have slipped so far down the drain that I couldn't have come back.

Start the conversation

Talking to someone is a brave and important step. Choose someone you feel comfortable with and tell them what's bothering you, what you're up against, and what you're really embarrassed or ashamed about. Choose someone who can listen well without judgment; someone who accepts you exactly as you are. First choice might be your partner, if you have one, but if you find that too difficult, choose a good friend, your sister, your mother, or that dear neighbour who always gives you good advice. Here are some conversation openers you could use:

- I don't need you to say anything, I just need you to listen to me until I'm finished talking.

- I haven't been feeling well lately and I think I need professional help.
- I have a problem that's been really bothering me, and I'd like to talk to you about it.
- Ever since I gave birth, I worry all the time and I don't know how to stop.

Maybe the other person will reach out and grab your hand or give you a hug. If you can, try and accept these warm and loving gestures. You deserve it so much.

Don't give up

One of my clients told me how she tried to explain her grey cloud to the people in her life. She noticed a lot of misunderstanding by her in-laws, especially her mother-in-law who reacted quite judgmentally. When my client indicated that motherhood was quite tough for her, her mother-in-law remarked, 'Yes, that's the way it is, suck it up and move on.' This really took my client off guard and discouraged her from speaking to anyone else. Eventually, a month later, my client dared to tell her husband she wasn't feeling well and that she believed she couldn't cope with motherhood at all. Fortunately, her husband reacted very kindly, was worried, and took her seriously. He asked her questions and showed understanding. Because of this, she felt able to tell him what was going on deeper inside her mind. Together, they started looking for help and they came to me.

Unhelpful reactions

Unfortunately, some people don't react with understanding or compassion. There isn't enough information out there about postpartum depression, and there is a great deal of ignorance and misinformation. The most well-meaning people might say the most unhelpful things. Here are some tips on how to deal with unpleasant remarks:

Be honest about how their comments made you feel, and share this afterward with your closest friends.

Some of you, like me, might also want to answer back. Sometimes I'd fight back like there was no tomorrow. I once said to my friend's neighbour (whom I'd only met once and who dared judge me for having PPD), 'Listen, I don't know who you think you're talking to. But PPD is not something I chose. If I could have had a choice, I would never *ever* choose this. This depression is something I wouldn't wish on anyone, so quit judging me.' But even if you don't want to be as confrontational, just know that you *can* say something, mama.

Remember that another person's opinion is not necessarily the truth. It quite often isn't, in fact, because they have limited information as to what you're going through. Remember, you don't need to do anything with unsolicited comments or advice; you *can* put them aside.

What helped me tremendously was lowering the bar for myself and accepting myself. No, I didn't always like the way I was thinking or feeling, but not fighting it or trying to run away from it helped me so much. Staying in the here and now, in the present, was a big part of that. Worrying about what had happened in the past or might happen in the future made me feel terrible. But as I learned more about mindfulness and how to stay present and grounded, I noticed I worried less. I also felt better about myself, about being a mother, and I slept better at night.

Another reason people might be unhelpful is that our loved ones can't stand to see us suffering. Their way of coping might be to just deny it's happening, or minimize it. 'Oh, you'll be all right after a good night's sleep.' Understanding that they're trying to protect themselves might help you to not be too adversely affected by their remarks.

This may all sound pretty simple but, often, it isn't. You've just had a baby, you're in survival mode, and you hardly have time to think about your thoughts and feelings. This may be more than you've ever had to cope with before. I know I sound like a broken record, but it's worth repeating: It is very important that you seek professional help. If you notice that the conversations with your friends don't help or your mental state deteriorates further, please call the doctor.

Professional help

If you recognize the symptoms described in chapter 2, or if intrusive thoughts are making you suffer, please call your GP or primary care physician, or talk to your health care visitor as soon as possible. This is the first step in getting professional help with your PPD.

Your GP/primary care physician will help you find the right mental health expert. When making your appointment, ask for extra time and tell your physician what's going through your mind *right now*. You can say that you think you have PPD and that you need help. List your symptoms. It can be really helpful to arrive with a few bullet points written down.

If you're having intrusions, please mention them. If you feel too ashamed to mention the content, you could just say that the thoughts really frighten you. Be as honest about what is going through your head and body as possible. Don't be tempted to downplay your symptoms; remember that your doctor is likely to have seen many, many other women go through very similar difficulties.

A good doctor will be understanding and reassuring and will talk you through the various treatment options, which might involve therapy, medication, or referral to a specialist.

If you feel that your doctor doesn't understand you, ask for another doctor in your practice. Don't give up! It is very important for you to have a kind, understanding doctor who can help you face this difficult period. Your doctor will write a referral letter to allow you to see a psychologist.

Waiting Lists

If you have been put on a long waiting list to see a psychologist, don't lose hope. Ask if there is any more immediate help you can get. Stress that you need help *right now*, not in six months. One option for immediate help is finding a therapist who specializes in postpartum depression, like me. Don't let geography be a barrier, either. Many therapists offer Skype sessions, and there are online courses and resources, too. Some things in life simply cannot be solved alone. If you're feeling too unwell to be proactive and research the kinds of available help, I completely sympathize. It's a cruel reality that the more help you need, the less likely it is that you'll feel able to ask for that help, particularly if the help isn't immediately available. I recommend telling a good friend that you're not able to do the necessary research, and could they look into options for you. Resources include national charities such as NCT in the United Kingdom, mental health charities, and specialized postpartum depression support hotlines. In New York, you can go to the Motherhood Centre. You can find support group for mothers, lactation consultation, individual therapy, or more intensive services to help you feel better. Please ask for help as soon as possible, and don't try to cope on your own.

The power of shame

Why do mothers find it so difficult to honestly share what they really think of motherhood? I find this astonishing; I don't understand why there's still a taboo about the subject of postpartum depression in the 21st century. Why don't women talk more openly about it? I would have benefitted greatly if I'd already heard about it from a friend who'd experienced it.

I think the silence around the subject mostly comes from shame—no woman wants to be labelled a 'bad mother'. Becoming a mother is a big deal, and the new role doesn't suit all moms instantly. Why should it? Sometimes you have to practice for a long time before it comes more naturally. There's nothing wrong with that. Let's now agree that we stop pretending that it's easy and admit to each other that, sometimes, it's very hard and not always fun. Can we be honest with each other from now on? Can we tell each other openly and honestly that sometimes we aren't floating on cloud nine after giving birth? That we sometimes want to palm off our baby onto our parents and that we sometimes feel reluctant to pick them up, or that we actually find breastfeeding awful but don't dare stop? Be honest and share it! You'll help someone else, I promise.

Gender disappointment

On the subject of shame, I think it's important to talk about something else that many parents might struggle with and also feel deeply ashamed about: feelings of disappointment at their baby's gender. Many parents are relaxed either way, and many parents secretly hope for a child of one gender or the other. Does this sound familiar: You had it all pictured in your head. You wanted a baby girl or boy so badly. When you finally have the 20 weeks scan, you discover the gender of your child and it's not what you were hoping for. You fake a smile and pretend to be thrilled, but you're feeling more disappointed than you could have ever imagined. You're suffering from gender disappointment. Stigma subject 2.0. No one talks about it because the thinking goes that you should be grateful to even *have* a baby.

According to Huffington Post[3], a quarter of British moms suffer from a degree of gender disappointment phase. The disappointment is a bitter pill to swallow, because none of these women ever expected to react this way. Some of them took a very long time to get pregnant in the first place. They know they should feel grateful to be having a baby, and these moms and dads feel guilty and ashamed for having such negative thoughts. A further 3 percent of moms said the gender disappointment affected their ability to bond with their child long-term, and 6 percent would consider flying abroad for gender selection IVF, which is currently illegal in the United Kingdom.

According to a UK poll run by a popular parenting website, mothers are twice as likely to want daughters over sons[2]. My friend Kathy told me, 'I feel so embarrassed, but I can't enjoy this pregnancy at all. The weirdest thing is I already have a girl. So why am I disappointed that my second child is a boy? I mean, it should be the best of both worlds. I shouldn't be feeling this way. It's absolutely horrible.' Her husband was very understanding and helped her through it. She had a lot of problems attaching to the pregnancy and therefore her baby. When she had an ultrasound, she didn't want to look at the screen and she wasn't interested in picking baby names, clothes, or even a nursery for her baby. Kathy's feelings of guilt and shame affected her mood greatly. She had a rough time until the delivery. When her baby was born, she felt fine right away. She told me, 'It was like all my worries disappeared.'

The study also revealed the most common reasons parents gave for wanting a child of a certain sex. The top reason for wanting girls were that girls stay closer to their parents when they grow up (41%), girls are more fun to dress up (40%), and girls are better behaved (7%).

The top reasons for wanting boys were that boys are easier (14%), boys are more fun to play with (9%), or cultural reasons (4%). Fascinating stuff!

I think one of the main reasons gender disappointment feels so painful is that the parent feels ashamed. They might also really worry that their thoughts and feelings will prevent them bonding with their baby. Thanks to oxytocin, the hormone produced by your brain during your labour, you can attach to your baby right away. And you might fall in love with your baby even though the gender disappointment phase made you fear you never would.

So trust your ability to love your baby. Some mothers don't fall in love with their child right away or feel a bond, but rest assured that in the end you *will* bond with your baby; sometimes it just needs time.

CHAPTER 4

Breast or Bottle: Your Call

Breast or bottle,
As long as you are
Feeding your baby
With love

Breastfeeding is a much-discussed topic in our society. When we were in America for a few months, I noticed a lot of slightly obsessive talk about breastfeeding—about all the benefits of breastfeeding and how superior this natural way of feeding was. I barely heard anyone talking about the disadvantages. First of all, I want to make it clear that I'm also in favour of breastfeeding, but (and this is a major *but*) only within the limits that are feasible for you. I don't think it's right that *all* new mothers should be pushed or even pressured into a pattern of nipple shields, pumping, and the whole enchilada. The way that breastfeeding is often regarded as the only 'correct' form of feeding seems completely over the top to me.

I believe that every mother has the right to choose how she wants to feed her child. Yes, a lot of research has been done on breastfeeding and its many benefits for the baby. But there are also disadvantages, such as the stress a mother experiences if her child doesn't get enough nutrition. Some babies don't latch on properly, some mothers produce milk that isn't enriched with all the normal nutrition but instead is watery, and some babies don't drink for long enough and never get to the hindmilk. (Hindmilk is the high-fat, high-calorie breast milk your baby gets toward the end of a feed. It's richer, thicker, and creamier than foremilk. This issue can happen if your breastfeeding doesn't get off to a good start.) In general, people don't speak openly about breastfeeding problems. Every mother who has just given birth wants to provide the very best for her child. In addition, the uncertainty that comes with being a new parent means that mothers can be particularly susceptible to the opinions of others, especially the women who belong to the 'breastfeeding mafia'. I think this is a rather heavy term, so I call them the breastfeeding gurus—that sounds a bit nicer.

A pregnant client once told me that she had already decided not to breastfeed. She didn't want any more demands on her body after giving birth and wanted her breasts to be hers and hers alone. I find this perfectly understandable. However, people in her immediate environment questioned her about it all the time: 'Wouldn't you like to at least try to breastfeed? It's said to be so good for your baby.' Once the baby was born and she was bottle feeding, complete strangers would ask her out of the blue, 'Why aren't you breastfeeding?' My client was completely disconcerted by this. On the one hand, she felt guilty, and on the other hand, she wondered why people weren't minding their own business.

Fiddling

I started breastfeeding right after giving birth to my oldest daughter because I felt that it was my moral duty (here we go again). I felt pressured by society, by the breastfeeding gurus. I felt as though giving my baby a bottle would mean I was failing as a mother. Why didn't I think for a moment, *What am I getting myself into? Is what's best for the baby, also best for me? Maybe I can bottle feed as well?* No, I felt I had to breastfeed. In retrospect, I don't understand why I was so rigid about it. But when I tried to breastfeed, the drops of colostrum came out with a lot of difficulty. I literally milked my chest with a shot glass under the pump, because that way we could measure if any milk was coming out at all—three full days of *fiddling*'! I remember this time well, our desperation mounting because our baby was losing too much weight and we were told she'd have to be admitted to hospital if she didn't gain weight soon. Her skin was continuing to turn yellow, something that should have already disappeared, and she also became a bit drowsy. I was horrified and so anxious. When I saw that of the six drops of colostrum I had managed to squeeze out with a lot of effort and pain, at least three drops had accidentally leaked into my shirt, I couldn't stop sobbing. I really bawled my eyes out. I was so upset that those three drops of milk went to waste, because my baby needed them so badly.

This is how I drove myself crazy. Fortunately, before I gave birth (back when I could think with a clear head), I bought a package of formula, just in case. That formula was our salvation, and I just gave it to my baby at night. I also kept on pumping during the nights. I was determined as hell. All the pumping finally paid off, because on day four after the delivery, my milk started to come in. It no longer seeped but spurted and, before I knew it, I could pump with bottles underneath the pump instead of those idiotic shot glasses. So off I went. Even though it was 'great' to be able to feed my child, 'great' was the last thing I was feeling, because I was in so much pain whenever she latched on. I know that many mothers experience this initially and then after half a minute the pain fades away; however, that wasn't the case for me. That stinging, intensely vicious pain stayed and some-times became even worse. *What is this?* I kept thinking, shocked. *Do all mothers hurt so much when breastfeeding their child, or am I the chosen one forced to suffer while all the other breastfeeding moms carry on blissfully?* When our midwife arrived with nipple shields, I even let myself be talked into those as well. Nipple shields can help a baby latch on better and drink more easily. I couldn't even handle water from the shower touching my nipples, they were *that* sensitive. You can probably imagine that when the nipple shield came off my nipples, it hurt so much I screamed and start-ed to cry again. Fun times.

I managed a total of three months of pumping and feeding my daughter. Three months with chest inflammation and extreme pain. Never again. With my second child, born over three years later, I bottle fed from the start. Yes, there will be people who call me selfish. Yes, there will be people who judge me and call me a bad mother. To these people I want to say, 'Live and let live.'

My American friend was more or less forced to breastfeed by her mother-in-law. When I heard this, the hairs on the back of my neck stood on end. Unfortunately, I hear many similar stories from my clients. Mothers, or mothers-in-law, foist themselves upon these new mothers with well-intentioned advice about breastfeeding. Even with the best intentions, because they often only want to 'help' their daughter (or daughter-in-law), they don't realize that their advice often has the opposite effect, and the mother in question starts to feel more insecure about her own capabilities as a mother. It seems like that was the case with my American friend. 'Once I switched to bottle-feeding,' she said, 'I hid the packs of formula food from my mother-in-law. In fact, I pretended it was expressed milk.' It was so sad to hear that she felt the need to disguise her own choices and lie about it, too. I think every mother should be free to make her own decisions without feeling the weight of the world's opinions on her shoulders. A new mother already has so much on her plate, let her be who she is and accept her choices. *Let it be.*

Facts and fictions about breastfeeding

When I was breastfeeding, I heard from many people that breastfeeding could help with postpartum depression. A Dutch website published a study by the University of Cambridge, which had conducted research among over 13,000 new mothers[4]. The findings showed that breastfeeding could even halve the risk of postpartum depression, that is, if all works properly and runs smoothly. But not if you experience a lot of pain and your child does not latch on properly. In the same article, they explained that if breastfeeding does not run smoothly, this can actually make the symptoms of postpartum depression worse. Not just that, but breastfeeding problems actually doubles the chance of postpartum depression occurring. In other words, if breastfeeding goes smoothly for you, there will be loads of benefits for you and your baby. If it doesn't go well, it can cause problems.

'The women who did want to breastfeed, but who did not succeed, eventually appeared to have the highest risk of postpartum depression of all the groups that were included in this study,' says researcher Maria Lacovou. Like many other mothers, I hadn't known that. This researcher recognises that 'it is, of course, wise to encourage women to breastfeed, because of all the benefits it has. But we must not forget to continue to pay attention to those women who are unable to breastfeed while they are so willing to do so. They have such an increased risk of postpartum depression, so it is wise for maternity nurses and other professionals to keep an eye on things.' Maria Lacovou also states in the article that the new mother's fear of failing in the eyes of society also contributes to her risk of mental health problems after childbirth.

Just a few months after giving birth, I read about the phenomenon D-MER (Dysphoric Milk Ejection Reflex), a condition that occurs in women who are breastfeeding. The symptoms involve experiencing such adverse emotions that breastfeeding becomes associated with very negative feelings. The moment the milk starts to flow freely toward the nipples, negative emotions are triggered—fear, anger, depressive feelings and restlessness—and can last for a few minutes. The good news is that the condition, which is caused by a disturbance of dopamine levels in the blood, can be treated. If you recognize these symptoms and think you may have D-MER, please check out the website d-mer.org.

Stop if you need to stop

If you add up all the evidence, women who aren't feeling mentally well after giving birth shouldn't be pushed into breastfeeding. I think nurses in maternity wards at hospitals, obstetricians, doctors, midwives, and health visitors who visit mothers at home should be specially trained to recognize all the signs of PPD. If you're a health care professional and you suspect that the mother in front of you suffers from PPD, please advise her to do what she feels is right, not what is expected of her by society, friends, family, or anyone else with an opinion on the matter. Unlike the women who think it should be illegal to not breastfeed, I would strongly advise women who are already depressed or who are genetically more at risk of developing depression to stop breastfeeding if it isn't going well. Don't get me wrong; I'm definitely not against breastfeeding and, if it's going well, I would advise you to continue with it, for all the benefits it provides you and your baby. But if you've been trying for a week and it's still not working or running smoothly, please stop. Or stop even earlier, if you notice signs of D-MER or you feel complete aversion to nursing. It's perfectly okay to stop. Really. Stop driving yourself mad. Stop pushing past your own limits. It isn't necessary. Children grow strong and healthy when fed with formula milk. They function perfectly well, and 20 later, no one asks your son or daughter whether or not they were breastfed. In fact, here in the Netherlands, the quality of our formula milk is so good the Chinese are importing it to China. Not too shabby.

The benefits of formula

Although there are many benefits to breastfeeding, formula also has a lot of pros. For example, it's full of vitamins. You have less stress about whether you're producing enough milk and whether your baby is short of any nutrients. Above all, you know exactly how much food your child is getting, because you can monitor his formula intake easily. Of course, this is also possible if you're pumping and giving your milk to your baby by bottle, but that does mean more work for you. During the three months I was breastfeeding, I lived the life of someone feeding twins.

Another advantage of bottle feeding is that your partner can do the night feed without you needing to pump, which gives them quality time with the baby, too. It also means that you can sleep through the night and rest up. Take a moment to let that sink in. You've just given birth, which has a major impact on your body and mind. You're exhausted, hormonal, and perhaps overwhelmed. You need time to rest and absorb the momentous change in your life.

Whether you opt for breast or formula (or both), it is solely up to you and your partner to decide, no one else. I just want to reiterate that I think breastfeeding is an excellent choice, but only if *you* make that choice. I recommend, if possible, talking through your decision with your partner before the birth, because afterward, you'll be a bit of a mess because of the hormones, lack of sleep, and so on, and making a rational decision is hard to do in those circumstances. You could for example say, 'We'll try breastfeeding for five days. If it doesn't work by then, we can switch to formula.' Have you already given birth? No problem, it's never too late to switch to formula.

A client once told me that she didn't dare stop breastfeeding. It wasn't going very well and she was feeling like a failure. I hear this a lot in my practice. So much emphasis is put on breastfeeding, and mothers feel a great sense of failure if it doesn't work out as they hoped. My client was pumping at work and hating it. At some point she had such a low supply of milk that after weighing the pros and cons, we agreed that she would stop. She was very happy with her decision. She suddenly had a lot more time for herself between the feeds, something she really enjoyed.

Meet in the middle

Of course, you can also choose the middle road by combining breast and formula and giving both to your child. There is a lot of talk about 'nipple confusion', that babies no longer want the breast once they've drunk from a bottle. There are ways you can help prevent this. For example, if you give your baby a bottle (in addition to breastfeeding), you should first gently rub the bottle over his lips, so he slowly gets used to the teat. He'll then search and latch on to the teat of the bottle. (That's how your baby latches on to breastfeed, as well. Your child searches calmly where the nipple is located, before latching on.) In this way, your baby will not become 'lazy' but will automatically look for the teat.

How do you combine breast and bottle? You can choose to breastfeed during the day and bottle feed at night. Or, if your milk hasn't come in yet after delivery, first give your baby some formula and then switch to breastfeeding. There are countless options. By combining bottle and breastfeeding, your child gets the best of both, and it also prevents him rejecting the bottle. As you can imagine, bottle rejection has the potential to cause problems later on, for example, if your child won't accept the bottle when at day care.

This flexible approach really suits many women who appreciate the benefits of both breastfeeding and bottle feeding. Whichever decision you make, it's always the right decision because *you* made it, both for your child and for you.

CHAPTER 5

How to Stop the Negative Spiral

Happiness is
Letting go of what
You think your life is
Supposed to look like
And celebrating it
For everything that it is

{ NOTE }

If you're depressed right now, I wouldn't start doing the mindfulness exercises outlined in this chapter right away. It's a bit like trying to walk on a broken ankle. Please get professional help immediately. The exercises in the book can then be practiced once you're under the care of a therapist or doctor.

All mothers worry. Especially at night. Clients often tell me that they're overwhelmed by an avalanche of negative thoughts as soon as they close their eyes. My advice is this: Allow the negative thoughts to just exist, without condemning them or judging yourself for having them, and then let them go. Easier said than done, I know. In this chapter, I'll give you tips on how to do it. Being able to recognize negative thoughts and live more consciously will be immensely helpful and can help break the draining negative spiral of worry thoughts and difficult emotions.

It sounds counterintuitive, but I promise you it's true: The thought is always there first, before the emotion. For example, you look in the mirror and your stomach is very puffy. The thought that pops into your head is, *My stomach is bigger than usual.* The feeling that follows is anger or sadness. But who says your belly is really bigger than usual? You, but are you objective when it comes to your own observations? No. When it comes to you, you're not neutral, so your observations are coloured by all kinds of negative thinking patterns and negative emotions. Practicing mindfulness can really help you stop engaging with the flow of negative thoughts. How? By learning to live consciously. What I mean by that is that you become aware of your thoughts, especially the negative thoughts. You learn to identify and accept them, instead of wanting to change yourself or fight against the emotions. For example, when I was in the midst of postpartum depression, I kept fighting the negative thoughts I had about myself as a mother. I did anything I could to prevent the thoughts popping up. It took all my energy and it didn't help at all. The thoughts just kept coming back. But once I accepted the thoughts in that present moment and then consciously let them go, I'd feel better within half an hour. That was so much more helpful than fighting the thoughts for hours and ending up in a negative spiral that could last for days, sometimes weeks or months.

If you try to suppress negative thoughts, they simply come back, even louder. Mindfulness is not passive resignation; it's like spreading your arms wide open to everything that comes your way, including the thoughts, conflicts, and emotions that you normally prefer to avoid. Bring it on! Mindfulness is about meeting your thoughts with curiosity, interest, and openness. It also includes commitment and compassion. If you're interested in something, you automatically pay attention. Isn't that great?

Mindfulness changed my life

When my therapist introduced me to mindfulness, I wasn't immediately enthusiastic. In fact, I thought it sounded very woolly and thought it was something for women with unshaved legs and Birkenstocks. Sorry ... Anyway, I wasn't immediately open to the practice, possibly due to my own ignorance. I look back to that time and laugh at myself, because mindfulness was the one thing that helped me through my depression the most.

After a few weeks of practice, it was like my blinders were taken off and I could finally see more clearly. One of my biggest discoveries was that postpartum depression wasn't my first depressive episode. I think I had a couple of episodes during my teenage years and college. If you've had an untreated depression, the chance that you'll suffer another depression at some point increases, unfortunately. The depression makes a connection in your brain between the gloom and the negative thoughts. This means that the normal discouragement every person sometimes feels can revive even stronger negative thoughts in your mind. It becomes a negative spiral that's hard to escape. Because I didn't know any of this, I kept falling back into negative episodes. So, when I lost my dear gran and had a traumatic birth, both triggered my PPD. It wasn't my fault. It was simply how my brain was structured by then. My brain worked but subconsciously had developed some glitches. Mindfulness made me understand this and made me live more consciously and aware of all the negative thoughts I would have during a day. And let me tell you, there were *a lot* of them.

Mindfulness was such a huge eye-opener that I began to spread the gospel to my girlfriends, and each and every one of them became converts. Because it has been so important to my own recovery, I've dedicated this somewhat longer chapter to getting you started on the path to mindfulness. I'll tell you how to recognize your negative thoughts, how to engage with them differently, and how you can experience more peace and openness through conscious living.

Your autopilot

Everybody does certain things on autopilot. Yes, you too! The autopilot allows your thoughts to wander off while you're engaged in a routine task. You're suddenly miles away from what you're actually doing. Suppose you have to post a letter somewhere on your way home from work. You drive home but you start to worry or daydream along the way. Before you know it, you're home but with that letter still sitting in your purse. Sound familiar? Your autopilot took over. The mental patterns that help us get stuck in a depressive episode operate in a similar way. They're old, ingrained patterns of thinking and behaviour, and they can suddenly take control. We surrender the wheel to the autopilot in our mind and thus create the conditions in which these subconscious mechanisms can do whatever they want. This always leads to the same negative feelings arising. How annoying is that?!

If you're often on autopilot (and therefore not living consciously), it makes you blind to other ways you could be living your life. In fact, it makes you blind to changes in general. I recently introduced the concept of mindfulness to a client who constantly worried that she was going to be fired from her job. Every day, she went to work with the world resting on her shoulders. She worried endlessly, day and night. That worrying led to dejection and depression. Then she began to judge herself for being so down and tearful, which of course only made things worse and made her worry more. She was caught in a downward spiral, which she wasn't able to get out of until she started applying mindfulness. She decided to throw herself into the practice of mindfulness after attending a workshop I gave. She became more aware of her negative thoughts as they popped up and then was able to let go of them. The thoughts no longer had so much power because she could see them for what they were: simply thoughts that brains constantly churn out, some far less helpful and truthful than others. This was such a huge relief for my client. After treatment, this lovely mom still e-mails me to tell me how she is able to apply mindfulness on a daily basis to all matters in her life.

Identify negative thoughts

Suppose you meet an acquaintance on the street. You greet them, but they don't say anything back to you. What's the first thing you think? *Why didn't she answer me? Is she ignoring me? Maybe she thinks I'm stupid or unimportant. In any case, not important enough to say hello.* Do you recognize this way of thinking or do you have a completely different version? Why did you think that thought at that particular moment? You could have thought, *Maybe she just didn't see me.* Why do you immediately jump to the worst possible interpretation? Why can't you trust that you're good enough just as you are? It's really you that gets yourself down. *Why can't I think like others? Why can't I trust that everything is good just as it is?* And there goes the negative flow of thoughts again, an endless stream of worry, a flood of thoughts and emotions that you can't stop. At least that's what you think.

But if you notice the initial thought, it can't run away with you. With mindfulness, you can break the pattern of one negative thought generating numerous others. You're no longer the victim of your negative thoughts. You are not your thoughts and vice versa. Remember that! Everyone has negative thoughts; it's just part of life.

I found it amazing that with a simple exercise such as the three-count breathing exercise, I could calm my thoughts. Without forcing it or having to put a lot of effort into it, my inner voice quietened down.

{ THREE-COUNT BREATHING }

I use this breathing exercise a lot, especially when I'm deep in the chaos of the morning or evening routine with my kids. Why? Because my kids drive me mad sometimes, and mommy doesn't want a mental breakdown. So, when they're throwing food or painting with ice cream on the windows (true story), I just close my eyes (or not, it's rather risky with a toddler in the house), and I do the following exercise, wherever I am.

Imagine you're at work and suddenly you feel very stressed because you still have a lot to do and you have to pick up your child(ren) from day care. This is the perfect opportunity to do this exercise. It goes like this:

- Find a room where you can be alone. Even the toilet is fine.
- Breathe in for 3 seconds and out for 3 seconds. Repeat this for at least 1 minute, or longer if you have time.
- Rest for a moment and feel the changes in your body.

Drifting away

Mindfulness can help you step aside from the flow of thoughts and look at what you actually feel at a certain moment. Zoom in on that feeling, and do it with curiosity and without judgment. Does it hurt? Don't be afraid of the pain; as soon as you breathe into it, the hold the feeling has over you loosens. All shall pass, and as soon as you realize that, you'll be so much freer. You don't have to think or have an opinion about any particular emotion. You just have to notice it and breathe. Sometimes it helped me to visualize the pain or discomfort and embrace it. No judgment, just letting it be there. It was already there, so why judge it? Why fight it? Just. Let. It. Be.

It felt very zen and soothing for me. It might sound strange, but believe me, it works. There's something comforting about knowing that nothing lasts forever. I didn't have to cling to any negative thoughts about myself anymore; I simply let them drift away. Find some imagery that works for you and use it time and time again to let your negative thoughts go. For one person, it might be a cloud that drifts away, while someone else might prefer a boat that sails away. I had a thought that just wouldn't leave me alone: *I am a bad mother*. I became obsessed with the thought. It was incredibly painful. My therapist said at one point, 'There's that negative thought again. Get rid of that thing, throw it over the fence! Out with the old, in with the new!' We both laughed. I found my own metaphor that helped me accept the negative thoughts and emotions and then I was able to let them go. My metaphor was a Moses basket, so I put my negative thought (*I'm a bad mother*) in that basket and let it drift away. Some thoughts were very persistent, taking a number of baskets before they left me alone. Sometimes, letting the basket float away down a river wasn't enough. Sometimes, I needed to let that Moses basket full of negative thoughts thunder down Niagara Falls. But eventually, the negative thoughts would subside, and I would finally get peace of mind.

Think of an image that works for you. Choose whatever feels good, and from now on, let every negative thought drift or float or sail away after you've addressed it and accepted it. Don't hold on to it! One of my clients who attended the mindfulness workshop said to me, 'I've learned to recognize earlier when I go on autopilot. I now know that I can stop and have to notice in that present moment what I'm really thinking or feeling. Mindfulness isn't woo-woo or only for spiritual people. I think it's logical and practical. If I have a lot of negative thoughts, I regularly blow them away in a cloud. I also try to be more aware of my activities, especially when I'm with my son.'

This mother's story is a good example of how mindfulness can work for you. Practice letting the cloud, balloon, basket drift away. Yes, it will take some practice. But just like learning to ride a bike, it gets easier.

Living in the present

Awareness prevents you going on autopilot, where old habits take over. Awareness allows you to recognize those old thinking habits for what they are. Eventually you'll even be able to see your worrying patterns from a distance, and perhaps even look at them with humour.

Living in the present moment is a good start. If you often think about situations in the past or the future, constantly rehearsing or rehashing, you're no longer present to the here and now. You become completely absorbed by your thoughts, and at that moment you really feel like you're actually in the past or future. You experience the emotions; you rehearse that event in the future or relive the emotions from the past. You experience thoughts and emotions relating to events that you've already left behind or that will never happen at all. No wonder you often feel miserable and bogged down with worries.

Simply 'being' in the here and now sounds easier than it actually is. But with practice, you'll really notice a difference. When you're in the mode of just being, you learn that you don't have to be anywhere else and you don't have to do anything other than what is needed at that very moment. Your mind can dedicate itself to the here and now, so you can be fully present in all that life has to offer you. This doesn't mean it's forbidden to think about the past or plan for the future. Of course not! It simply means that when you're doing something, you want to be aware that you're doing it.

The raisin exercise is a classic mindfulness exercise and one of the first steps to a higher level of consciousness.

{ THE RAISIN EXERCISE (IN BRIEF) }

You look at the raisin first and smell it. Really pay attention to how it looks and smells. If you want to put it in your mouth right away, please don't do it yet and be mindful about this excercise. After looking at it and smelling it for a while, slowly explore it with your lips and tongue. Then put it in your mouth and chew it very slowly. It might feel strange to chew so slowly, but do it anyway. You'll become very aware of taste and texture. This exercise can take a couple of minutes.

Believe me: every mother who does the raisin exercise for the first time is very surprised at the structure of that little fruit that she normally eats a handful at a time. I know all mothers are super busy and sometimes will feel as though they don't have time for practicing mindfulness. But I really encourage you to make time for it. If you want to live a more mindful life, invest in these little exercises on a daily basis. You'll soon notice a difference.

Conscious attention

How can you live more consciously in the here and now? First, you consciously pay attention to what you actually experience when you're engaged in routine tasks. Each day, approach one task with the same level of attention as you gave the raisin in the exercise. The point is to pay attention in a gentle way to what you are actually doing at that moment. Try to be as aware as possible in a nonjudgmental way. Be kind to yourself. Many people who start practicing mindfulness for the first time think it's almost impossible to keep your full attention on the smallest things, such as brushing your teeth. Often, they don't like doing it at all and find it evokes aversion and irritation. They think of every-thing except brushing their teeth. It's all very frustrating and, as your to-do lists grow longer and your baby starts crying, it can feel like an inefficient use of time. But truly, it's not.

Be gentle with yourself; mindfulness requires practice and it will not happen immediately. Just try again the next day and the day after. Just keep going. There are benefits, even if you only notice yourself being mindful for a fraction of a second at first. Every time you notice yourself getting distracted, gently bring your mind back to what you're doing. The more you notice that your mind has wandered, the more you're practicing mindfulness. Give yourself a compliment when you succeed.

Have you seen your baby look at her hand? Completely mesmerized and completely absorbed in the moment, she stares at her own small fist. So cute! She watches her own little fingers, her nails, the folds in her skin—she's very much in the moment. And the good news is that you can do this as well. Our minds have a natural innate ability to do it; we just need to train ourselves. One of the easiest exercises to start with is to focus your attention on one object. Your attention will wander off, and when it does, you just gently bring it back. Full instructions follow.

Research has shown that this practice is very effective at helping calm the mind. How does it work, exactly? Imagine that you look at a fire and you only concentrate on the flames. At that moment, your brain activates the network that only needs to focus on those flames, and everything else fades away. You end up in 'being mode'. At the same time, a different brain network is inhibited, the one that distracts you by thinking of other things you should be doing right now—the 'doing mode'. All this happens without you having to force it. It's as if your brain is lighting up your chosen object and darkening everything else. This exercise is a friendly, gentle way to calm your mind under any circumstances. It's very different to deliberately forcing yourself to stop thinking about something, or trying to banish certain thoughts. I can almost hear you think, *I'm a tired, busy, working mom with a crying baby on my arm. I don't have time to stare at a candle*. But I'm here to tell you that you can do this exercise at any moment of the day. So put your baby to bed, switch off your phone, and do it anyway.

Use your breath to help anchor you, letting it gently flow in and out of your body. Become aware of the changes in your body as you do this exercise.

{ FULL FOCUS }

Choose an item that appeals to you, something that has no emotional charge. Go look at it for a minute. If you find a minute too long, start with 30 seconds. You can use a timer but use a gentle one. You don't want to jump into the air with shock when it goes off. Then all your good work would vanish into thin air. Try the exercise without an alarm, and do it until you feel it has been long enough. Just follow your intuition. The duration of the exercise is not important. The goal is to keep bringing your mind back to the object of focus.

For example, light a candle and gaze into the flame as if it were the first time you'd ever seen fire. You'll notice the effect of your full focus. Maybe not right away; you might need some practice. But please keep practicing, as eventually it will feel more comfortable and less awkward. Your mind will calm down at some point, so be kind to yourself and don't judge yourself if it doesn't work right away. The exercise is a beginning to a more enlightened and more conscious life, and you deserve it. Nobody wants to worry the rest of her life, right? If you find yourself doing 1 minute without difficulty, you can extend the exercise to 5 minutes.

Affirmations

What many mothers notice when they get into mindfulness is that they are more relaxed and if they get a negative thought, they soon recognize it. *Aha! Here's that thought again. I already know that one and I don't need to do anything with it. Everything's fine, exactly as it is.* If you keep repeating this, it becomes automatic. I did, and I advise you to do the same. Think of a few powerful sentences that you can repeat the moment a negative thought comes up; for example, *I don't have to check anything, everything is good, just as it is.* I use positive affirmations every day. If necessary, write your positive affirmations in a notebook so you can remind yourself of them when necessary. That helped me enormously. At some point, your brain picks it up and you won't have to check the notebook anymore. Affirmations can be said in your head or spoken out loud. Sometimes I said them in front of a mirror and found that very powerful. You can also write your affirmations on post-its and stick those throughout your house, so wherever you go, you're reminded that everything is fine, exactly as it is. That you are good, exactly as you are.

Become aware of your avoidant behaviour

No one likes feeling bad. When negativity sets in, we all want to avoid the feelings at any cost. You might not be aware of your efforts to avoid your emotions, thoughts, feelings, and body sensations, because they can turn into addictive habits. Those cookies you have to have after you speak to your mother on the phone, for example. Be honest, you'd prefer to avoid negative feelings if you've had painful experiences in the past, right? You can pretend that the negative feeling isn't there, but actually that is exactly the same as pretending that you don't hear that crazy ticking sound in your car engine when you drive at 100 miles an hour, which is a very effective way to ensure that your engine fails a few miles down the road!

If you suffer from depression, anxiety, or emotional dysregulation, it's possible that you may be someone who ignores or suppresses their emotions. If you shut yourself off from the sensations that occur in your body from your thoughts and emotions, it's likely that you may eventually crash. Bearing in mind the longer-term side effects, pushing away and avoiding thoughts and feelings is not the way to deal with difficult situations. If you try and repress emotions, they will eventually erupt to the surface. That happened to me. I tried to push down my intrusive thoughts as much as I could. I felt so ashamed and guilty that I was thinking about how I could push my daughter off a bridge in her pram. I didn't know what to do with myself. So I pushed those thoughts away, instead of addressing and accepting them in the present moment, but suppressing them only made me feel more and more anxious and depressed, and I got into a vicious cycle I couldn't get out of.

How can you learn to tune in to your thoughts and feelings again without being immediately overwhelmed by them? The downward spiral of negative feelings often starts with a physical response. Instead of repressing thoughts and feelings, we should learn to pay attention to our physical sensations. Do you feel a weird vibe in your lower abdomen? Do you have painful shoulders? Do you suddenly get a stabbing pain in your head? Very good! You already noticed them and are recognizing your standard reactions. You just stopped the succession of negative thoughts. Awesome! As with the other exercises in this chapter, learning to pay attention to your physical sensations takes a lot of practice. Start by regularly practicing the body scan exercise that follows. You'll soon find you're starting to recognize signals from your body much more frequently.

Body scan

The book *The Mindful Way Through Depression: Freeing Yourself from Chronic Unhappiness* is full of really helpful exercises that helped me learn how to start feeling more in tune with my body. One of my favourite exercises is the body scan, which teaches you how to explore your body bit by bit. You'll learn to recognize pain sensations and muscle tension.

Imagine this scenario: In a meeting earlier, your boss told you a few things that you don't agree with. You've been grumpy all day but don't know (yet) where your grumpiness actually comes from because you're constantly in 'doing mode'. The tension you experience toward your boss feels like a cramping sensation somewhere in your body. If you noticed this cramping, you may ask yourself, *Why do I have a stomach ache? Why is this happening right now? Could it have something to do with the situation with my boss?* You might have had other experiences in the past where stress also manifested itself as stomach ache. You've already experienced this! So instead of ruminating on how angry you are with your boss, notice how and where you're feeling tension in your body, and see if you can nonjudgmentally become aware of those feelings. Accept how you're feeling and let the negative thoughts and emotions go, using your own chosen metaphor. You've just taken a huge step.

{ *THE BODY SCAN IN BRIEF* }

Sit quietly in a chair or lie down and close your eyes. Put your hands in your lap. Breathe in and out. Starting with your toes, gently pay attention to what is going on in them. After a few moments on the toes, proceed to the next body part. Maybe the arch of your foot. Then your ankle. From your little toes to the top of your head, simply scan each part of your body. Open your eyes when you feel ready.

The body scan will help you become more aware of everything happening in your body and mind. The body scan is about focusing on the physical sensation, thus preventing you chasing after negative thoughts or fighting against anything that makes you feel uncomfortable.

Your inner barometer

Our feelings come in many different intensities. Our inner barometer, like an actual barometer that continuously monitors atmospheric pressure, gives us information about the atmosphere inside our head. You can consult your inner barometer at any time of day to become more and more aware of what's going on inside your mind. This ultimately ensures that you can understand yourself better and feel more stable in difficult situations. Learning to read your internal barometer doesn't just happen overnight, so treat yourself kindly.

The internal barometer is basically a meter that tells you how you're *really* feeling inside. It is not the outside version that says 'I'm fine' twenty times a day. Not, it's the real you, with the real, raw, and unfiltered feelings you can have on a daily basis. I had no idea I had an internal barometer, but when I discovered it, it really helped prevent me getting into that negative spiral of emotions. It was such a revelation that I made a promise to myself to check in with myself, with my state of mind, three times a day. Was my state of mind positive or neutral? Whatever it was, I just moved on with my day. If it was negative, I thought about what I could do to help myself in that moment. I'd excuse myself and pop to the toilet, for example. Or if I had people over, I'd go upstairs to our bedroom and practice one of the mindfulness exercises I've outlined here.

Continuing the journey

Mindfulness not only helped me in my recovery from PPD, but it has helped me live a happier, fuller life, too. I've said it before, and I'll say it again: I really encourage you to commit to practicing these exercises for a few seconds or minutes every day. This has just been a brief introduction to the subject of mindfulness, and I've listed some of my favourite books on the topic below, so you can delve deeper if you wish.

I see how many mothers benefit from mindfulness and how it helps them get out of their depression. When you're in the deepest darkest depths of depression, the light seems so far away, but mindfulness makes you feel like you've just come up for a big breath of fresh air. It feels so liberating, and I want you to experience it as well. I hope that in this chapter I've explained the benefits of mindfulness and I hope it offers you just as much peace and relief as it has brought me. Good luck!

Further Reading

Mindfulness: In the Maelstrom of Life by Edel Maex

The Mindful Way Through Depression: Freeing Yourself from Chronic Unhappiness by Mark Williams, John Teasdale, Zindel Segal and Jon Kabat-Zinn

CHAPTER 6

When Sleep Deprivation Has Taken Over Your Life

Mombie:
A sleep-deprived supermom
who feeds on caffeine and survives
on sticky kisses and messy smiles,
Mombies are master multitaskers
And suck-it-uppers

Sleeping is a hot topic for many new mothers. You want nothing more than to just sleep, but it can be virtually impossible in the first few months. Or longer. You get well-intentioned advice such as 'You have to sleep when the baby is sleeping.' I always wondered, *Do I have to cook when the baby is cooking, or clean when the baby is cleaning?* I mean, I really had more stuff to do than just sleeping. Most mothers have a huge to-do list. Yet, despite all our other tasks, it is very important to get as much rest as possible. You just became a mother, which is a big experience that can hit you pretty hard. Whether it was a fast and 'easy' delivery (is there such a thing?) or a long and intense birth, you have to recover, both mentally and physically. Your body has to heal, but your mind has to recover as well, by processing what you went through. Add that on top of an enormous rolechange, along with all the uncertainties that maternity entails, and you have a very challenging scenario that encourages fulltime worrying.

You might find yourself worrying a lot, not only during the day but also at night, perhaps especially at night, when your child finally is asleep, but just when you want to start your well-deserved night's rest, here come those thoughts again. Not all the thoughts are negative; some can start off quite innocently. You're thinking about how nice it was to see your friend today and have some coffee and cake together. How great it was to introduce your baby to her. *Right…I had cake…* Before you know it, you're off: *I ate too much. Maybe I shouldn't have had dessert. Crap, I'll have gained five pounds tomorrow. Shit. Maybe I should work out tomorrow. I don't have time! And anyway, I don't feel like working out. Is it already two a.m.? And I'm still not asleep? Dang it! I'll be so tired again tomorrow. I really don't want to be so tired all the time. I have to sleep. Please, let me just fall asleep.* And on and on.

No mother wants this. Fortunately, there's a way out.

Mindfulness is the solution

Mindfulness can be practiced every day of your life, both during the day and at night. For example, if after the umpteenth sleepless night, your child starts crying, your first reaction might be, *Nooooo! Are you hungry again? I really don't want to get out of bed, I just want to sleep.* One of my clients told me that she would get angry at night when her baby cried 'again'. Whether her baby was hungry or needed a nappy change, my client would be furious. 'I just lay in my bed and waited until my baby started to cry. That way I was still awake when it happened. Because once I'm asleep, I can't wake up that easily anymore,' she confided.

Do you recognize this? What if you approach that negative thought about being awake at night with curiosity instead of condemnation? See what happens. Where do you feel the irritation in your body? Where does it manifest? Breathe slowly into that place and let it go. Do you remember the metaphor exercise? Please do that. Put that negative thought or emotion in a balloon or boat or basket and let it drift away. Accept that you sometimes feel dejected. Don't judge yourself for getting angry because your baby was hungry. Deep inside, you know as well as I do that you're not angry with your baby; you just feel desperate because you're so incredibly tired, which is very understandable. Once you've allowed that negative thought to drift away, see if you can bring yourself into the present moment. What's happening around you? If you're feeding your child, can you notice things about your baby that delight you? Perhaps the baby is perfectly content in his own happy place. He doesn't worry whether or not he's drinking his bottle in the right way or whether he's opening his mouth enough. You were born the exact same way. You used to be someone who didn't worry about how you should think or feel about things; you didn't judge yourself. By applying mindfulness to your life, you can find that peace of mind again.

Surviving periods of sleep deprivation

The bad news is that there is no magic solution to the problem of sleep deprivation. The good news is there are quite a few tips and tricks to help get you through this really intense period. For some, this period lasts 'only' a month or so. For other parents, it takes up to a year or even longer. Read on for my top tips.

Nutrition

I cannot stress this enough: Your engine needs fuel. Fill it up as lovingly as you can every single day. Three meals a day and regular snacks. Chocolate is indispensable to me when I'm very tired, because (a) I've earned it, and (b) I've earned it. Drink 1½ to 2 litres of water a day. I love bananas and eat one every day. They give me significantly more energy than other fruit. I also add nuts to my meals, because the omega 3 fats in them are so good for the body.

Exercise

I'll cover this more in the next section, but exercise deserves a brief mention here. Moving around really helped me a lot. That sounds a bit counterintuitive, because who has the energy or wants to work out when you're exhausted? Yet the endorphins released through exercise really boosted my mood and actually gave me more energy. It was also great to do something for myself and to give myself a short break from doing laundry or worrying about my baby and my lack of sleep. I'm not telling you to work out seven days a week at the gym—far from it. I'd go for a walk most days. I'd stroll around the neighbourhood or walk into the city to meet a friend, instead of taking public transportation or my car. I love to cycle, so I'd do that when my babies were bigger and could sit in their bike seats. They loved it too, because there's so much to see. In the Netherlands, our kids sit on the front side of our bikes when they're little. You can watch them, and they can see everything that's happening in front of them. And you can give them kisses on their head if you have to wait at a traffic light. Both my girls loved it so much and still do. I loved being outside and it also helped me tremendously in my recovery from my PPD.

Routine

Try to keep your day and night routines as regular as possible. Everyone will have different advice about this, so I can only share what worked for me. Go to bed as early as possible. Don't wait to see if your baby still wants a bottle at 11 p.m.; just go to sleep. Your baby might ask for that bottle at 1.00 a.m. and then you will at least have had a few hours sleep. Every minute of sleep is a win, if you ask me. During the day it's essential to get as much daylight as possible. It helps your body clock reset, and the sunlight will recharge you a bit.

Appearance

I looked terrifying in the mornings. I was so freaking tired, I could barely put one foot in front of the other. I'd look into the mirror and wonder what had happened to my face. I'd have major bags under my eyes and have a puffy face like you wouldn't believe. I also had red spots all over and seriously thought I was getting pimples again. The horror! This happened with both my babies.

The sleep deprivation aspect of having a newborn was the hardest part for me. Not just because I looked horrible, but also because it made me feel very wobbly and out of balance. One small thing that helped was to take a bit of time for myself first thing. In the mornings, I would attack my face with a nourishing day cream and some serious eye cream. Then I charged at the bags under my eyes with concealer, because otherwise I looked like a raccoon. A beautiful outfit also cheered me up enormously, because if I look nice on the outside, I feel a lot better on the inside, too. Wherever I found a coffee machine, I'd sit next to (or preferably in) it. I can't live without caffeine during intense periods without sleep. A friend of mine likes a powernap at her desk, or she'd sometimes nip to the loo for a quick nap. If you're desperate, shut the door behind you and lean into that powernap. Desperate times call for desperate measures.

{ QUICK SLEEP TIPS FOR PARENTS }

- Switch your phone to night mode from 7 p.m. This makes the light less bright and the colours on your screen change to sepia tones.
- Provide a lot of light during the day; this keeps your natural biorhythms intact.
- Dim the lights in your living room; this promotes the production of melatonin.
- Put your phone, laptop, or tablet away two hours before you want to go to sleep, in order to stimulate melatonin production so you fall asleep faster.
- Open the window in your bedroom; you'll sleep better with fresh air.
- Don't leave your phone next to your bed, because electromagnetic radiation can disturb your sleep.
- Drink less alcohol and caffeine (full disclosure: I can't follow my own tips; I love my coffee too much!).
- Take melatonin if you really can't sleep. This substance is also made by your body and helps you fall asleep more quickly and also sleep through the night.

Sleeping through the night

Sleeping through the night is another hot topic among new parents. Your baby will not sleep through the night on her own straight away. She will need guidance and gentle encouragement to do so. I'm no baby whisperer or anything like that, so I'll simply tell you what I've read about the subject and what I did with both our girls.

A baby develops her own biorhythm in the womb during pregnancy, meaning that she'll have her own personal wake-up and sleep rhythm. Often your baby sleeps during the day, lulled into sleep by your everyday movements. Swinging back and forth in mom's belly is very blissful. I almost fall asleep just thinking about it. At night, however, she'll wake up because you're not moving. I often felt a lot of moving and kicking in the evening when I'd crashed on the couch, and sometimes it would wake me from a sound sleep in the middle of the night.

The schedule your baby has developed inside your womb is likely to continue in the first period after birth, which means that during the day she will most likely sleep constantly between meals and be awake a lot during the night. Obviously you're not going to immediately reverse this routine once your baby is born. It's frustrating and tiring, but my advice is to give it time.

When your baby is about six weeks old, she's likely to be able to sleep for stretches of up to six hours without waking up. That long stretch is a godsend if you're sleep deprived and exhausted, so you'll want that long stretch to happen at night rather than during the day. There is a saying: 'Never wake a sleeping baby'. I disagree. If you wake your baby every three hours for a feed during the day you (a) make sure she gets enough food intake and doesn't have to make up for that at night, and (b) your long stretch of sleep will happen at night. My husband and I started the three-hour routine between 0–2 weeks postpartum. You can start this routine whenever you feel ready or comfortable, regardless of whether you're breastfeeding or bottle feeding. There are many books available that can guide you, but this is how we did it. It took a little time for our babies to get used to the three-hour routine, but after two weeks, they were settled. They knew the deal was eat, sleep, poop, repeat. I'd wake them at 7 a.m. if they weren't awake yet and I'd change their diaper, dress them, and then feed them. After that, there was playtime. I know this might sound crazy, because how can a newborn play? But we'd put them in the pack-and-play and lay toys around them that made noises and turn the musical mobile on.

A newborn tends not to stay awake for longer than an hour at a time. So I'd put them to bed an hour after waking up. I'd also tell them what was happening, such as 'You're going to play now and after that you'll go to bed and sleep.' When I was swaddling them, I would tell them, 'It's time for sleep. Mommy will be close by and I'm always here for you.' When they slept, I knew I had about an hour for myself, so I'd shower or clean the house, rinse some bottles, etc. With my second child, I learned that I could also use that time to watch some Netflix! The house would still be messy an hour later, so why not use that hour to recharge? This routine also makes sure your baby learns to fall asleep without a bottle or breast. Because you keep your baby awake between the feed and his or her nap. Some babies won't fall asleep without mommy's breast or the bottle and moms get so exhausted at some point. The routine teaches them how to sleep on their own, which also later on in their little lives is a huge help and relief for the parents.

This routine made the whole day clear for all of us. For example, when we wanted to visit family, we knew the best time to leave (not during feed time) and when we wanted to be back home. We made sure we were back in time for the evening routine that always started at 7 p.m. The routine therefore lasted from 7 a.m. to 7 p.m., and during the waking times it was fun, lights on, playtime, singing songs, and so on. But when evening came, we wanted to make it as boring as possible, because babies need to learn the difference between day (fun) and night (boring), meaning they learn that it's hardly worth waking up at night. This was our evening routine: bath, playing the same song, diaper on, jammies on, and feeding at 7 p.m. We'd dim the lights and minimize talking. I also avoided eye contact when I could because I wanted to show my girls that there was no more play or fun time today. I found it difficult at first, but after a few weeks it became easier. After the feed, I'd burp them and then swaddle them. I'd sing a Dutch lullaby and clearly say goodnight. Or as we say in Dutch, 'Slaap lekker.' I'd switch the lights off and leave the room. Both babies would fall fast asleep soon after that. As I mentioned, it took them a couple of weeks to get used to the routine, but after that it was easy peasy. I also recommend a night feed at 11 p.m. This way, you prevent the six-hour sleep stretch happening too early, while you're still awake, and you also give them more food, which helps them sleep through the night. People call this the dream feed because your baby will hardly seem awake, but she's awake enough to drink, even if she has her eyes closed the whole time. Keep the lights dimmed, don't talk too much, and if she needs a diaper change, do it before the feed, so when she's topped up with milk, she can fall asleep easily and won't wake up from the diaper change.

After the dream feed you let her sleep until she wakes up for a feed. This might be between 2 a.m. and 4 a.m. Once you've noticed that she woke up at the same time for three nights, for example at 3 a.m., you set the base time as 3 a.m. You won't feed her before that, because you now know she can sleep that long.

You can now start gradually stretching the base time by 15 minutes every three to five nights. This is how we did it: When our girls woke up we would first wait for five minutes to see if they'd fall asleep again or not. If you're not comfortable with five minutes, start with one minute, then two, three, etc. We'd let them know we were there but that it wasn't feeding time yet. They call this 'spaced soothing.' We'd stroke their forehead or temple, put a hand on their chest, and whisper 'shhhh'. You don't do this to shush them; the 'shhhh' noise resembles the noise they hear in your womb, which is calming and makes them feel safe. You can also use the spaced soothing technique during the day, to help your baby fall asleep on her own. If at any point you feel like your baby is too upset, pick her up and cuddle her, of course. I always used it as a last resort but trust me, there were nights when I was walking around the room with a crying baby and wondering how I was ever going to pull this sleeping through the night thing off.

Gradually, we stretched the middle of the night feed from 3 a.m. to 7 a.m. by extending the time of the feed by 15 minutes every three to five nights, using the spaced soothing technique. It sometimes happened very fast, nudging the time forward by 30 minutes, but we also had nights when they went backward and we thought we'd lose our sh***. Both our girls were sleeping from 11 p.m. to 7 a.m. when they were about nine weeks old. We dropped the 11 p.m. feed when they were 12 weeks old. I found that incredibly scary, but the books told us they were ready, so we just did it and voilà! Of course, this takes hard work and effort. You have to be consistent in your actions and do it every night, otherwise it probably won't work. And it's easier to get in place when babies are very young, rather than doing it when they're six months old. I'm not saying it's impossible when they're older, I'm just saying it'll take you a little longer to get there. Don't let yourself be stopped by that. Sleep is the greatest gift, after all. For your baby, but also for you. I remember the first time Liv slept through the night. I woke up in the morning and thought, *She didn't cry?* I woke my husband and asked him if he'd gone to her in the night. 'Nope.' Of course, I had a major freak out and leapt out of bed and rushed into her room, where she was peacefully lying there, looking at me with her beautiful eyes like she was saying, 'Hi, Mom, what's up?'

Getting babies into a sleep routine is not always easy and sometimes we were close to despair. There were many nights that I rocked my babies in my arms who were screaming because it wasn't feeding time yet. I felt guilty, of course, but teaching them how to sleep through the night is a great gift you can give your kids. Kids who sleep better through the night are even thought to make better students.

Nobody gets happier or is more enjoyable to be around when they haven't slept for a few nights (let alone a few months). Getting a baby into a good wake-sleep routine can be quite tough, but it's definitely worth it.

Maybe you're reading this and feeling annoyed, thinking, *Yes, well, I tried this but it didn't work for my baby.* I feel you! It's so frustrating when you're doing the best you can and it seemingly isn't working out. I urge you to give it another go. And try to stick to the routine every day (not changing it every other day). Make a plan that you and your partner feel comfortable with and stick with it for at least three weeks; it's likely you'll see a big difference. Add another four weeks, and your baby will be a happy camper, too. But ultimately, as I repeat throughout the book, you need to do what feels right for you and your family. With a bit of experimentation, you'll be able to find your own method that suits you best.

Let your child stay overnight with your parents

If you can, give yourself a baby-free night as a treat. Call in a favour with your parents or in-laws and see if they'd be willing to host a sleepover. It can be immensely beneficial for you and your partner, and your child grows used to being around other people. Ask your parents, brother, sister, friends. They might really love spending so much time with their grandchild/nephew/niece/godparent.

My neighbours were a lovely older couple who had recently retired. They adored Livia and our neighbour Lous baby-sat her weekly. When she offered to take Livia for the night, I felt hesitant at first. Could I impose on them like that? When she insisted that she'd love our baby girl to stay overnight and didn't mind having to get up, I caved. Liv slept blissfully happy, and so did we. No alarm clock, no crying baby—almost as it used to be.

If the sleepover goes well, you could even consider taking the next step and going away together for an entire weekend to fully recharge. But only do that if you're really up for it. I wasn't ready until Livia was two years old. When we had Emmi, my husband and I went away together without our kids when she was a year old. So, it got easier for me. Having a weekend as a couple again was wonderful. I can highly recommend it. We had so much fun together, lunching, enjoying a good glass of wine, taking powernaps (so needed), and walking around Rome. We couldn't believe how much time we had now that we didn't have to dress/feed/change anybody else. It was a revelation, and we plan to do it every year now. Let's see if we can pull that one off, shall we?

Swaddle your baby

A lot has been said and done regarding swaddling. Some people are against the practice because they believe a baby shouldn't be restricted from moving. Others say it's the best way to let your baby sleep. I'm one of those people. I love swaddling. I did it with both my kids and felt it was a life saver. Imagine this: You're a baby and you've lived in your mother's womb for nine months where it was warm and cozy, the noises were soft, and you could touch all the 'walls' 24/7. Besides that, there wasn't a lot of light or stimuli. Then you're born. Lights everywhere. Huge open spaces. Lots of things happening. You know that moment right before you fall asleep and you suddenly feel like you're falling off a building and jerk? It's called the startle reflex. Your baby has that startle reflex, too, and right before he falls asleep, he can easily get startled by any kind of stimulus, a loud noise, or even his own hands moving. He starts to cry because he's scared and doesn't want to fall asleep on his own anymore. Swaddling can solve the problem.

There are a wide range of swaddle cloths available, some that hold the baby really tightly and others that fit a bit more loosely. The looser ones are fine when the baby is small. But once he's reached the three-month mark, he'll struggle his way out of them. I preferred the tighter swaddle cloths. And we noticed a massive difference with both our girls when we first swaddled them: During daytime naps and at night, they fell asleep way faster and slept longer. As a parent, you should always do what feels right for you and your child, but don't worry about harming your baby by swaddling him. You won't!

Sleeping in shifts

As a new mother, your body has already had to endure a lot. Give your body the opportunity to heal by taking as much rest as possible. I often advise new parents to sleep in shifts in order to make sure you and your partner both get as much sleep as possible. You can do this by agreeing, for example, that your partner does the last bottle at 11 p.m. and that you do the night feed at about 3 a.m. It's absolutely pointless for both of you to get up. Decide who does which feed and make sure the other person can sleep well. Some mothers automatically wake up when their baby starts crying, even though they know their partner is going to do the feed. If this happens to you, sleep with earplugs! Or if there is somewhere else that's out of earshot, the partner not 'on duty' can sleep there.

If you bottle feed your baby, your partner can just as easily do the night feed as you, even if it may not feel that way. When you're breastfeeding, you might need to pump later at night to avoid waking up with engorged and painful breasts. See what time is most convenient for you. I, for example, pumped at 10 p.m. (or sometimes at 9) and then I could sleep till 3 or 4 a.m. As a mother, you'll sometimes feel like you're the one doing all the tasks. Remember, you and your partner are in this together, so asking them to do a night feed means you trust them to do it. And while they do, you can get some serious hours of much-needed sleep.

You cannot function without sleep

There's a reason the CIA uses sleep deprivation as a method of torture. Sleep deprivation is awful. You can learn to recognize your fellow sleep-deprived parents: Just look for the women repeatedly visiting the coffee machine, or the woman in the supermarket with dark purple bags under her eyes.

As I said, sleeping in shifts is a godsend. Some mothers don't like it because it means having to go to bed very early in the evening. My advice is to try and get used to it. Get as many hours of sleep as you can. This is going to save you. because once you've slept six consecutive hours, you'll feel like a whole different person. A six-hour night can honestly feel as if you've slept until noon, especially if you've had only a maximum of three hours of sleep a night during the previous weeks.

Your cognitive functions increase sharply once you've slept well. You'll be able to concentrate much better and for longer. In addition, your memory recovers, your perspective changes, and it's easier to think more clearly. So, if you're reading this and your baby is sleeping and the laundry is folded, the groceries are done, and you have the time, put this book down and take a nice long nap. Actually, take a nap even if the groceries aren't done and the laundry isn't folded!

If, however, you're reading this and your baby is screaming, it's going to be okay. He won't scream forever, I promise. Try to go outside for a walk. Your baby might fall asleep and you can enjoy the silence and the fresh air. I know this first period postpartum is hard. Very hard. You're a good mother, and it does get easier.

CHAPTER 7

Start Moving and Get Outdoors

*Exercise not only changes your body,
it changes your mind,
your posture,
and your mood*

This chapter is all about how exercise can help you mentally. But I think it's important to note that despite all the fantastic benefits exercise brings to your mood, it can be a tricky subject. It's linked to how we think we look, and it can become yet another thing we beat ourselves up about. After my first child, I felt very self-conscious about my body. I had a big wound down under and those stitches made me cry out with pain every time I needed to get up or go to the bathroom. I also expected to lose weight way faster than I actually did. I kept looking at my 'wobbly' stomach, and criticising myself harshly over it not being flat yet.

My therapist recommended exercise as being good for my mood, but I sometimes focused too much on losing weight instead of feeling good. I don't know why I was so mean to myself, but it certainly didn't help me at all. Writing this, it makes me want to go back to the old Tilda and give her a hug, telling the old me that everything will be okay and that weight or body size isn't really that important and that loving yourself is vital. I think we women should be a lot nicer to ourselves. We shouldn't be punishing or judging ourselves. Size is just a number. It doesn't define you. Not at all. Perhaps because of what I learned through having PPD, I've become a warrior for self-love in the last couple of years. I feel that loving yourself unconditionally is the key to true happiness.

That being said, I felt very unhappy after giving birth, and mentally I was all over the place. I never would have guessed that exercise would help me so much in my recovery. After only about three months of working out again, I started feeling much better. However, if you've just given birth, you shouldn't be thinking about working out right away. You'll want the thumbs up from a professional first, and most mothers want to get to know their baby and develop a routine before leaping into the gym.

In an amazing and perhaps counterintuitive way, physical activity can be very mindful. As soon as you get into the groove of what you're doing, you can't worry or overthink. While you're paying attention to what you're doing, you don't have time to have negative thoughts or feelings because you're focusing on that barbell in your hands or that yoga pose you're trying to balance in. I still love to work out, because it helps me to de-stress, calm down and unwind.

If you're feeling low after childbirth, the last thing you probably feel like doing is exercise. Once you're physically ready, however, I really recommend making exercise part of your own routine. First, it will give you some much-needed alone time. Second, those endorphins generated by exercise are so helpful in elevating mood. Still not convinced? The third reason to exercise is that it is a fantastic way to practice mindfulness.

The link between exercise and mood

Most of us know that exercising is good for us. Not just for the body but also for the mind, and that's what I'm mostly interested in here. During exercise, endorphins are released, and they give you that blissful feeling. But if you're depressed, you don't feel like doing anything, you feel chronically tired, and lacing up your trainers probably seems beyond you. Still, my therapist advised me to work out as often as I could bring myself to. If that wasn't do-able, she advised me to at least go for a walk outside with my baby. Not only does fresh air improve your mood, but the endorphins that are released during a simple walk will also do you good.

Because I didn't take antidepressants, it took me longer than average to get over my postpartum depression. But I felt much better because of the exercise. Of course, I also had days where I was completely done with it all: the depression, the negativity, the crying. And on days like that I really didn't have the strength for a workout, so I'd go outside and take my baby for a walk. We had a nice park near our house and a lot of people would be there walking their dogs. Liv really liked looking at the dogs, and when she got older, she wanted to pat them and would then laugh. Other times I'd put her in her bike seat and I'd cycle anywhere I fancied. Feeling the wind on my face, breathing in the fresh air, made me feel better instantly. Liv loved seeing new sights and people and would stretch her little arms toward everything she wanted to touch. I'd lean over and kiss her on her head and smell her hair. Because it helped me so much, I gently encourage you to find an activity that works for you, even when you feel down. Keep going, even when you don't feel like it. Be kind to yourself and reward yourself when you've done it.

The benefits of working out

As I just mentioned, exercising helps with depressive symptoms, but it has even more advantages. A physically active person learns to recognize and trust their body's reactions. Over time you can push your limits, if you want to, which will increase your self-confidence. The fear of setbacks and failures decreases. In turn, feeling more positive makes you more able to cope with daily activities. If you have postpartum depression, exercising interrupts the vicious and negative cycle. For example, I discovered a sense of independence and pride when I worked out. It was a feeling I hadn't felt in a very long time. The pride came from the fact that after all I had been through—the intense and traumatic delivery, losing my grandmother—I was still here, doing my best as a mother and in the gym. It made me feel proud that my body was able to recover so well and that I could build up my physical strength. There can be a social aspect to exercising, too. If you go to the gym, say, at the same time each week, you'll start recognizing people, maybe even having the odd chat. Even the briefest social encounter is beneficial and will help you feel less isolated.

The positive psychological effects don't lie. People with depression are often trapped by clinging to beliefs that are far from rational. I, too, had the cruellest thoughts about myself: *I'm a bad mother. I'm constantly failing.* I saw these negative thoughts confirmed everywhere. I also manufactured arguments as to why I shouldn't go running, such as, *It's raining and I don't want to get wet* (ever heard of sweat?), *I'm too tired, I can't do this* (you'll be tired for the rest of the year so you might as well go), etc. But because my therapist encouraged me to exercise, I mostly did it anyway. It helped having someone hold me accountable. And once I started noticing the benefits, I wanted to keep going.

If you exercise outside, there are further advantages. Women who have just given birth or who have PPD will have experienced disruption to their circadian rhythms, otherwise known as your bodyclock going haywire. Getting outside and getting some sunlight can really help reset those biorhythms. In addition, research shows that being outside in a green environment has a positive effect on mood.

So put this book aside, download a map on your phone, and start walking. Please build it up slowly. Even if you just go outside for a few minutes, that's fantastic. You might think about trying a phone app, which can be motivational. For example, I used MapMyRun, but a client of mine liked running with an audio programme on her phone. I also hear good stories about the Runtastic app. All three have the same thing in common: They motivate you to go running and moving and, more importantly, *stay* running.

What to expect

When you start exercising for the first time after delivery, there's a high chance you'll lose some urine. Not huge puddles, but a decent amount of dripping. I felt very embarrassed when it happened. The advice of a pelvic floor physiotherapist is to insert a tampon before you exercise; it will close off your urethra a little so you won't leak as much. Or you can use a pad; you'll feel safe and if you experience urine loss, your (sports) pants will at least remain dry. Experiment with exercising at different times of day, if you can. I found there was much less leaking in the morning than in the evening. It's important to build up your workouts slowly but steadily, and don't push yourself too hard in the beginning. Give your body the chance to get used to physical activity again.

If you're not a Sporty Spice

Whether we're mothers or not, lots of us need a bit of encouragement when it comes to committing to a regular exercise routine.

And for mothers, it's even harder because you're constantly tired and the nights with little sleep take their toll, so it's understandable that you want to lie on the couch and binge on Netflix. Figure out the best time of day for you to exercise. You might choose to start moving during the day, because your energy level is higher and you know that at night, when your baby is asleep, you can relax. Whatever time you choose doesn't matter, as long as you feel good about it.

Consider trying one of the apps I mentioned earlier, to keep track of your progress. I personally enjoyed seeing how much progress I was making. It kept me motivated and was quite fun, but I also was just happy to get out of the house. Another benefit of working out was that during it, I wasn't thinking about all my responsibilities. I didn't have to think about my endless to-do list. I was just Tilda enjoying my workout. Nothing more, nothing less. It felt liberating.

You might enjoy exercising with a friend. You're much less likely to cancel your yoga class if you know your friend will be there in the studio, relying on you to turn up so you can suffer though those downward dogs together. Plus, working out with a friend doubles up as a nice opportunity to socialise and to catch your breath, away from all things baby related.

If you have a partner, perhaps you can work out a timetable where you take it in turns to look after the baby while one of you heads out the door (to the gym, to see a friend—it's all good). Beg a favour from friends or neighbours if hiring a babysitter for a couple of hours isn't an option. You'd be surprised by how many people find looking after a sweet baby for 90 minutes is really quite fun. Maybe you can team up with another mom, and once a week you look after each other's baby so one of you gets the chance to go to a blissful candlelit Body Balance class, or whatever it is that floats your boat. There are also gyms with day care, which makes it even easier to go work out.

Healing from negative body image

As a teenager I struggled with an eating disorder. I only completely overcame it recently, by learning how to accept myself just the way I am. I remember punishing myself for eating too much and forcing myself to go on the treadmill for an hour. Working out was often a tool to compensate for the binges I'd had. It often felt like punishment rather than a pleasure. It wasn't the kind of role model I wanted to be for my daughters. I got scared. What if my girls got an eating disorder, too? What if they didn't want to eat because Mommy was constantly freaking out about food or gaining weight? What if they started judging themselves for having a certain body size or shape? No! I didn't want any of that to happen. I wanted my girls to feel proud of their bodies. And I wanted them to see a proud mom embracing her curves and loving herself unconditionally.

When I found Jessi Jean on Instagram, she was a revelation to me. Through her masterclasses and podcast, she teaches women all over the world how to love themselves and how to empower their bodies and souls. She told me and all the other women in her online group that the weight loss industry has been making billions by giving us the impression that fat is wrong and that we should all conform to some kind of skinny standard. That if you're not a certain size you don't count and that you have to be skinny to fit in. I followed her online programme and gradually learned how to love myself unconditionally. Yes, it was hard. I'd binged all my life and used food to manage my emotions. But I haven't binged for a year and a half now and have truly found food freedom. I work out now because I want to, not because I feel I have to. I feel working out is empowering. I'm honouring my body by keeping it healthy and fuelling it when it needs to be fed and working out so I can sprint beside my girls without getting short of breath, not because I want to overcompensate for what I've eaten or shouldn't have eaten.

After finishing Jessi Jean's programme, I felt like I could finally be a good example for my girls. I've always told them that they're beautiful inside and out. Our oldest is very bright and sensitive. One day, she came home telling me that a kid in school called her fat. She was clearly upset. I told her that 'fat' is a word only narrow-minded people use and that we don't say stuff like that in our house. I told her that a person is so much more than just their body shape. For example, smart, creative, sweet, loving, and caring. A couple of weeks later our neighbour came by the house. He is 89 years old and said something about a fat cat that was playing in our yard. Liv quickly replied, 'We don't say fat in this house. You can't say that, it isn't nice.' My heart leapt. I couldn't have been prouder of her, despite my elderly neighbour's confusion.

Relationship between nutrition and depression

There is a relationship between diet and depression. According to Mark van Essen, a varied and complete diet can prevent depression. Research shows that our Western diet, often rich in processed foods, increases the risk of depression by almost

60 percent. On the other hand, healthy food can lower the risk of depression by 26 percent. Mark also adds that sugar consumption is characterized as one of the major causes of depression. This is because sugar and processed foods cause inflammation in your joints and contribute to depressive feelings. If you have postpartum depression, you often have a deficiency of vitamins B6, B11, and B12. A deficiency of omega 3 fatty acids can also cause depression. Vitamin supplements can be helpful, but it is even better to get all your nutrients from your regular food intake. I try to stick to fresh foods and not use processed foods too much. I'm no Martha Stewart, so I choose to cook simply but efficiently—fresh veggies and lots of casseroles.

Helpful diet for postpartum depression

Protein-rich food is very good for you and makes you feel fuller for longer. Examples of protein-rich foods include:

tuna	mackerel	trout	mussels
turkey	chicken	beef	game
eggs	goat's milk	snow peas	green beans
peas	lentils	chickpeas	walnuts
cashews	hazelnuts	Brazil nuts	pumpkin seeds
pine nuts	linseed	sesame seeds	mushrooms

It's also important to consume **healthy carbohydrates**, such as:

apricots	blackberries	raspberries	mango
peaches	figs	grapefruit	currants
endive	asparagus	beets	broccoli
zucchini	sprouts	carrots	kale
green cabbage	red cabbage	garlic	alfalfa
parsley	cocoa	honey	millet
buckwheat	basmati rice	oats	rye

Fats get a lot of bad press, but they are vital to your health. Choose good sources of fat, such as:

extra-virgin olive oil	coconut oil	palm oil
hazelnut oil	walnut oil	

Also make sure you include **vitamin B–rich products**, such as:

potatoes	grain products	bread
meat	dairy products	

Foods to limit or avoid (temporarily):

sugar	alcohol	refined food	ready-to-eat meals
pork	liver	smoked sausage	cheese
anchovy	sardines	shrimp	salmon
sauerkraut	spinach	tomato	avocado
pineapple	kiwi	strawberries	ice cream
vanilla	cinnamon	raw fish	

Processed foods are full of omega 6, which you want to avoid.

Do what feels right for you

Recovering from childbirth isn't a walk in the park. As I've said before, your body has been through a lot. Give it time to heal. Pushing yourself into a military sports regime won't help you and most likely will make things worse. Be as kind to yourself as you can possibly be. Working out is good for you, if you do it for the right reasons and not because you want to fit in or measure up to the weight loss industry's marketing strategies. You don't have to be a size zero to matter. You *do* matter, as a person, always.

If you do decide you want to work out, do it because it helps you feel physically stronger and more powerful and because it helps you recover from PPD[5]. Thanks to the endorphins, the feel-good chemicals, you'll start to feel better again. There's something for everybody: Some women like yoga or Body Balance, whereas other women prefer running or HIIT (high intensity interval training), to get that cardio buzz. There's always the good old free weight workout you can do on your own, or try a class such as Bodypump or Zumba, if motivation is harder for you. The social aspect really spoke to me. I could kill two birds with one stone: work out and have fun!

The Things Nobody Tells You

Those other moms
Don't have a clue either

There are certain things in life, and in motherhood in particular, that nobody talks about—the embarrassing or awkward stuff that people don't like thinking about, let alone talking about. If you're bold enough to talk about it, other mothers will say, 'Oh yes, that happened to me.' But why didn't they warn you? For example, I wish someone had told me how important it is to be stitched up right away after giving birth if you had an episiotomy or a tear. Because if they wait for an hour and a half (as happened to me), you no longer have adrenaline rushing through your blood and you feel EVERYTHING. They can't numb that area, so for many women, the stitching sometimes is worse than the actual labour.

I often wondered why nobody told me about things like this before I had children. After two kids, I now have a theory. Most mothers are embarrassed to talk about it. For some reason this stuff is taboo. I realized later that I'm a rarity in being really open about all the postpartum stuff. Like peeing my pants, or how I screamed at the midwife who stitched me up without anaesthetics. I seriously wanted to slap her. Plus, I think women worry about maybe putting off would-be mothers. I still advocate for more openness. Every woman about to have a baby (or thinking about having one) deserves to know what might be in store. I know I would have loved to know way more up front. I would have been more prepared. I know not everyone wants to talk about all the excruciating details of the birth or the period after, but let's make a deal, okay? Let's agree that we're no longer pretending that giving birth or being a mother is all nice and easy, and that some things about becoming a mother or going through labour are freaking hard. Let's be more open about the challenges we face as mothers and that it isn't like you see in the movies, TV series, or social media. Let's. Keep. It. Real.

For example, I didn't know that after women have given birth, they can still experience contractions. These can last for an entire month, multiple times a day, mostly when the baby is latching on during breastfeeding. Also, if you had a long delivery and you had to push for over an hour, you might become (temporarily) incontinent. I didn't know any of this until I became a mother, and honestly, I felt screwed over by Mother Nature and by other women who hadn't told me. So, this chapter is full of the things I would have found helpful to know beforehand. I'm not giving you the information to scare you, but to give you what you need to know before, during, and after labour.

Asking for an epidural

In the Netherlands, not everyone gives birth in a hospital. Many women deliver their babies at home with a midwife and sometimes with a doula. But if you do give birth in a hospital, it's good to know that every major hospital has an anaesthesiologist on call 24/7. So don't hesitate to ask for an epidural during your delivery if you want one. In my country, some older nurses will try to talk a woman out of an epidural, but if you want one, insist upon getting one. If you can barely talk through painful contractions, your partner can advocate for you. A morphine pump is also an option. This provides relief but is not nearly as strong as the epidural. Please do your research ahead of time and work out what you want in terms of pain relief during the birth. Don't be afraid to stand up for yourself and don't be put off by a healthcare professional who is against pain relief. You're the one going through it, and therefore you're the one who gets to make decisions about your body.

If you get an epidural, you'll also receive a urine catheter, just in case. As though the labour itself isn't fun enough! The epidural numbs any signals that you need to pee, which is why you get the catheter, which empties your bladder. This is included in the epidural service, free of charge. For me, it was set up before I got the epidural. I asked for it to be the other way around, but that wasn't possible. No, it wasn't fun, but it was bearable.

Normally, the catheter will be removed immediately after birth, unless—like me—you stay admitted for the next 24 hours. In that case, they let the catheter sit for a while because you officially have to urinate within two hours after the catheter has been removed. Unsurprisingly, most women don't want to do this, two hours after pushing a watermelon through a keyhole. If you can't pee within those two hours, the catheter has to be replaced, and believe me, you really don't want that to happen. So drink as much fluid as you can and make sure you pee within those two hours.

Thankfully, giving birth is not just pain and suffering. I found it one of the most beautiful, inspiring, and impressive experiences of my life. You have a mission: You're going to push your child out with every power you have in you. You leave behind the woman you once were and will never be again. *You're not just Tilda now, you're also a mother,* I told myself. It is very impressive to see how far your own body can go to get your baby out. There is a primal force that will overwhelm you and at the same time encourage you. Be guided by that intense feeling, and surrender to it. There's no point in resisting it; your baby is coming out, regardless, so let those labour pains do their work and go with it.

Your vagina

Many women need help getting the baby out, for example if the baby's head gets stuck. If that occurs, the ob-gyn or midwife may decide to make a cut—an episiotomy. If that doesn't take place, you can tear. That sounds horrible, but it does have a small silver lining. A tear in your vagina heals faster than a cut because the ragged edges of a tear reattach and heal more easily than a sharp cut. According to my doctor friend, this is why an episiotomy is only done if it's medically necessary, for example if the child's heart rate drops too much during the pushing stage, or if a vacuum pump is needed. I had an episiotomy and was 'delighted' to have it. After pushing for two hours, I was starting to believe my baby was stuck down there. So when the midwife said she was going to do an episiotomy, I was like, Please, do it! NOW! Get her out! I didn't feel anything, because she did it during a contraction. In the Netherlands, they shut off the epidural during the pushing stage, which I find outrageous. I hadn't felt any pain for 20 out of the 22 hours, until they shut my epidural off. Then I was in so much pain. I hated my midwife for doing that. After the cut, I started to push again. Finally, my baby's head came out. I could feel myself tear a little, which later appeared to be a tear from the cut. Anyway, the episiotomy really helped me get my baby out and I was happy they did it.

The pain of both a cut or a tear can last for up to two weeks (or longer), then it really diminishes. It's different for everyone, but my advice is to let it heal before you even take a peek. I'm probably going to get a lot of criticism from midwives, maternity nurses, doctors, and so on for saying that, but I'm convinced that nobody is going to be happy to see the havoc down under during a period that is already intense enough. Wait until the six-week check up with your doctor or midwife and then take a look to see how you've healed. Or not, because that's fine, too. I kept on being asked whether I wanted to look at my own foof. I really, REALLY didn't want to. I was scared out of my mind about what I'd see. I mean, I was already mentally unstable. Did I really need another traumatic experience? No! I don't know why my midwife was so insistent about me looking at my *vagine*, but I was definitely done with her asking me if I wanted to have a look. At some point, I wanted to scream, 'Nooooooo! I. DON'T. WANT. TO. LOOK. AT. MY. EXPLODED. VAGINA!'

On the other hand, it might look better down there than you think and therefore be reassuring. So, if you can handle it, grab a pocket mirror and take a peek. I absolutely didn't want to look, but when I had my six-week check-up they asked me again and I looked and thought it looked fine. Fine. I had no other word. It wasn't as bad as I'd feared, but it did look blue and bruised. I could see the line from the episiotomy. It felt weird, looking at that scar. I felt vulnerable. I remember thinking, *Wow, this scar will never go away*. Until recently I'd still feel occasional pain in that scar area, especially around the time of my period. I try to see it as my battle scar now. Something to be proud of. Because I did deliver a baby, and what could make someone prouder than that, right?

'No, your vagina will never be like it was before.' That's what a midwife said to me. Really? Thanks. Awesome. Couldn't you guys have told me that in advance? And what does that even mean? I don't know how my vagina looked like before I had kids. It wasn't like I walked around with a hand mirror and looked down under every chance I got. I think she meant the way my foof feels or looks. She told me about normal vaginal tightness and how mine would now feel a little looser, something many women experience. I hated this talk, honestly. I felt as though someone had robbed me of my perfectly normal vagina. In the end, though, it wasn't so bad. I still enjoy sex and I'm happy with the situation down under.

Stitches are b*tches

I already mentioned how suturing must be done as quickly as possible after delivery, but I'll say it again now: Make sure you get any necessary stitches immediately after your placenta and everything else has come out.

I didn't get them immediately, because after I finished my 22-hour delivery in the hospital, my midwife suddenly vanished. I thought she might have gotten hungry or thirsty and was getting coffee. Or wine. Lord knows, I could have used some of that as well. So I wasn't alarmed. I lay in bed, legs still in the stirrups, cocooning with my miracle baby. Then I began to wonder where she'd gone. A new midwife arrived. Apparently, they'd just switched over shifts, the fourth shift of nurses and doctors I had seen coming and going during my labour. So my midwife wasn't just getting a cup of tea? No, she'd gone to do her paperwork so she could go home on time. She told me this herself later, when we ran into her as I was being transferred to my overnight room. It was understandable on one hand. On the other hand, the adrenaline that helped my body through labour had worn off by the time I got stitched up. Without anaesthesia. Because according to current expert opinion, anaesthesia doesn't help. I got a squirt of perineal spray over my war zone and just had to deal with it. It took half an hour. While I was being stitched up, my husband was doing skin to skin with Livia and couldn't hold my hand. At some point he offered me his foot to squeeze. I'm pretty sure I almost broke it. And I screamed. A lot. Please, state in your birth plan and agree beforehand that you want the epidural still on until you're all stitched up. Ask your partner to pay close attention that they leave it on.

Don't allow yourself to be dismissed or ignored. Make sure you aren't left alone before your vagina has been sewn up, if it needs it. You can just say this or ask them to help you right away. As a patient, you have the right to stand up for yourself and say what you want and don't want, even though it may feel as if the distance between you and an entire medical team is huge. Discuss this with your birth partner beforehand so they can advocate for you and make sure you're taken care of properly. Stand up for yourself, through your own voice or that of your partner.

Pee in the shower

Many women are afraid of urinating after giving birth, because everything down under hurts. Urinating usually hurts after delivery, it's true, but peeing in the shower is a great way to do it because the water thins the urine and lessens the sting. Just go nice and easy and don't think about it too much. And, who knows, you might be able to pee painlessly.

Peri bottle

When I gave birth, there weren't a lot of products I could buy for the postpartum period. Luckily, only five years later, there are plenty of options. I love the brand Frida Mom. (I promise this isn't an ad!) I simply adore the brand for their down-to-earth approach and wide range of inventive and useful postpartum products. My personal faves are the 'gown for when it all goes down' and the 'peri bottle.' The peri bottle is meant to relieve your foof while urinating, to avoid another ring of fire. To use it, you fill the bottle with water and squirt the water over yourself while peeing. I didn't have one when I gave birth for the first time, unfortunately. I had to be inventive; I used a measuring jug from my kitchen. A week later I used that same measuring jug for making lasagne sauce. It's a multifunctional jug.

Your first night as a mother

After your labour starts, you probably won't sleep for two nights in a row. The first night, because for some reason, childbirth often begins at night. And the second night, because you tend not to sleep after a birth. No, you don't sleep at all. My night nurse told me, 'No, sweetheart, no one is sleeping in these rooms. They're all recovering and resting, but sleeping, no.' After the birth, I started sweating enormously at night. Puddles of sweat in my neck, between my breasts, and on my back. I placed a towel and a clean shirt on my bedside table every night, so I could dry myself and change before doing a night feed. I didn't want to be shivering with cold while feeding my baby. These night sweats will stop as soon as your hormones rebalance. Nothing lasts forever.

The bags you grow under your eyes in the weeks after the birth are hardcore! Mine were darker than Dutch liquorice. The golden tip is this: If you really have to leave the house, buy a good concealer. Fatigue starts to hit in a big way. Your ability to concentrate drops to a historic low. You'll probably notice that you can no longer read instructions properly. None of this matters at all, as it too will pass. You just have to go through it. My mantra was and still is: It's a phase. That works every time.

Stowage in your breasts

Milk production often starts after a few hours and sometimes within one or two days after delivery. Because your body is preparing to breastfeed, more blood flows to your breasts. This means your breasts might become quite swollen and painful. This is called stowage. You can develop hard, sore spots in your breasts, and you might get a fever, too.

There's already a lot written about stowage, and there are all sorts of ways of relieving the discomfort. Crushed cabbage leaves in your bra or cold compresses against your breasts during and after feeding can help. Even mothers who are not breastfeeding will go through this, after a few days. A friend of mine who was not breastfeeding had massive boobs on day three after the delivery, and that was pretty painful. I worked through my engorged breast phase as well as I could, but it really hurt; I could barely sleep on my side. I grew to a double F bra size and had impressive veins that ran over my breasts and enormous nipples. My aureolas were the size of shackle discs and very dark. My breasts have remained half a cup size larger than my original size, and my nipples are back to normal, so don't worry, your boobs will be fine.

Meconium and intestinal cramps

It can take a few days before your baby's digestive system starts to work and she can poop. The time it takes varies from baby to baby. I believe it was our second night at home when shit hit the fan. Our poor girl screamed and screamed. She went completely ballistic. She cried for hours, and at the end of the night we no longer knew what to do. Even my husband, who is a surgeon and is normally super relaxed, started to get really stressed. He shouted something like, 'This isn't normal, is it? What should we do now?' Like I had a clue.

The diapers filled up quickly and became fuller and fuller, and what was in them looked nothing like human poop. It was a tar-like substance called meconium. It takes a lot of effort for your baby to work it all out and the pain that comes with it is no joke. We saw through that night, rocking our little girl and comforting her as much as we could, and later found out that her distress was due to her intestines working out all the 'mud' that was in there. This black sludgy meconium consists of swallowed hair, amniotic fluid, and other goodies that your baby ingested while growing in your womb. By the time breastfeeding (or bottle feeding) has started and your baby's gastrointestinal tract is filled with milk, these nasty cramps will decrease a little. To be subsequently restarted by new cramps, this time caused by gas caused by the milk. Newborns can find it difficult to get that air out, which means stomach pain. Sometimes they relieve themselves with an enormous fart.

I ordered Sabsimplex[6] drops on the advice of our friends. These are drops you can buy over the counter in German pharmacies and that simply and effectively merge all the little bubbles in milk (both in formula and breast milk) into one big bubble, making it easier for your baby to work the bubble out in the form of a huge burp or fart. The product has been around for 35 years and is reliable and very effective against intestinal cramps. There are plenty of things that seem to make the first three months of your baby's life difficult. Don't let cramps be one of them.

Postpartum contractions

Postpartum contractions are also seldom talked about, which is quite strange, given that every woman who gives birth has them. The frequency and intensity of the contractions will vary from mother to mother. Postpartum contractions have a useful function, ensuring that the uterus returns to its normal size and position behind the pubic bone.

Postpartum contractions can occur within an hour after delivery and can last for a month or longer. If you haven't been forewarned that you'll experience them, the pain can come as a nasty and alarming surprise. During these contractions, blood clots can come out of your vagina. These clots can sometimes be quite large, about the size of an orange. What's happening is that your womb is cleaning itself out from the inside. Very smart, but unfortunately often quite painful, the pain varying from a stabbing pain in your lower abdomen or lower back to something that resembles labour pains.

These contractions often begin once you're breastfeeding, but they can occur at any moment after childbirth. Unfortunately, unlike during birth, you don't have the benefit of adrenaline, so these postpartum contractions can feel very intense. It's all part of the birth circus, the postpartum period that's boosted with gifts, presents, love, and an extra gift called postpartum contractions. You can call your ob-gyn or midwife for reassurance, but rest assured that the contractions will subside, usually within a week or two.

Pooping for the first time after birth

This can be quite an experience. You'll be warned about it from all sides: medical staff, nurses, friends, you name it. It was actually a very easy experience for me, perhaps because I eat a lot of fibre-rich food and drink a lot of water. On day five postpartum (I checked the maternity report), everything finally got going. The fear is that your fresh wound will tear open again or your stitches will pop out, but that won't happen. Remember, you don't poop with your vagina but with your anus—a completely different area. So don't worry about it too much. I said, 'People, turn up the music a little, I think I'm going to poop.' That made my husband and the maternity nurse laugh so hard that I chuckled hard, too, and before I knew it, the ball dropped, so to speak. Use magnesium or a stool softening product, such as Movicolon, to make pooping easier. Breathe in (through your mouth, not your nose) and let it all happen. You've already given birth, so anything else really is a piece of cake.

Haemorrhoids

Haemorrhoids are another amazing gift you may receive. Many women report feeling like a baboon after giving birth. Haemorrhoids occur because there's so much pressure on your bottom while you're pushing the baby out. Haemorrhoids can vary in shape, size, and colour, but they have two things in common: They hurt and they can make sitting uncomfortable. There are products you can buy to reduce the size of the haemorrhoids, and you can look for a special ring cushion to make sitting more comfortable.

Take it super easy

Because your foof is quite painful those first few days (or up to two weeks) after childbirth, do whatever you need to be as comfortable as possible. Maybe this means a lot of lying down in bed, which puts the least amount of pressure on your pelvic floor. Any visitors can simply sit by your bedside or put a chair next to your bed. Many mothers can't sit comfortably on a chair because of the pain of the stitches (or haemorrhoids), but still they put on a brave face and sit with their visitors in the living room, smiling on the outside but crying on the inside. Don't do that, dear mothers! Listen to your body and stay in bed when you're in pain or tired. If you feel really good, there is of course nothing wrong with getting up and sitting in the living room. But if you're suffering, please stay comfy in your bed. You'll be up soon enough.

Incontinence

Nobody told me that sometimes you have to start months of pelvic floor physiotherapy after childbirth. Many mothers have problems like this after delivery. No matter how good your physical condition was before the birth, every woman can experience pelvic floor problems and suffer from incontinence. If the muscles of your pelvic floor are weakened during childbirth, it can be difficult to keep your bladder closed, which means that you'll have trouble holding in your pee. This also applies to the rectum; if weakened pelvic floor muscles can't properly close the sphincter, you can lose stools.

I was a kind of walking waterworks after giving birth. I continuously lost drops down under and sometimes more than that. For example, if I had to sprint to catch the train, or if I laughed uncontrollably, it would happen. I literally peed my pants every day. I couldn't run after my kids, or to catch a train, without having to change my underwear. I carried clean panties with me everywhere I went. I even peed during sex at one point. I thought it was terrible. Incontinence is the last thing you want to worry about, and some women are reluctant to discuss it with their partner. Trust me, I know. I felt so embarrassed I couldn't even talk to my husband about it. When I finally told him, his response was very sweet. He accompanied me to the doctor where I was delighted to discover that there were options for me. My advice is to speak to a doctor if incontinence becomes a real problem and interferes with your life. Although they won't necessarily be able to cure it completely, there are a range of options.

TVT stands for tension-free vaginal tape. TVT supports the urethra, which is the tube that carries urine from the bladder to outside the body. I decided to try it. I had the procedure done after giving birth to my second baby. I had to wait until she was 10 months old, and I also had to be sure that I didn't want any more kids. The surgery took 15 minutes. After I woke up, my groin was painful. I was able to leave hospital the day after the surgery and was back on my feet the week after. The first time I did a workout without peeing my pants, I almost cried with relief. Normally I would have had to change not only my undies but also my jeans or leggings. Now, nothing. Nothing! No leakage! None!

I know incontinence is embarrassing and you don't want anyone to know about it. Please know that you don't have to live with it for the rest of your life. Trust me when I tell you that the TVT procedure improved my quality of life *hugely*. Don't wait until you're 65 (true story from my ob-gyn). Talk to your doctor as soon as you can.

Your story

As we've established, you're not always going to feel super positive and intensely happy after childbirth. That's completely normal. You're exhausted mentally and physically and you have to process the experience. You'll be overwhelmed by love and responsibility for your little baby, and sometimes completely confused. Tell me about it! As soon as you can, just start talking, to a close friend, to your mother if you have that kind of relationship, to your partner, and the processing will start faster. We'll go into this more in the next chapter.

The pain (and for some, the trauma) of delivering a baby is not easily forgotten. Some say you forget all about it as soon as you hold your baby. But that isn't always the case and that's okay. Whether it was an 'easy' birth, a quick one, or one that lasted three days, every mother I know remembers the experience vividly, and some find it really helpful to talk about it. Some even try to outdo each other with their stories, but that's a completely different subject!

Birth trauma

Many mothers who come to my practice have had a tough or negative birth experience. I rarely speak to women who found it a piece of cake. (I find that such a strange expression, because what does it mean? And what kind of cake?) Of course, such women do exist, and sometimes the delivery goes smoothly. This section is for the mothers who had a tougher time.

If I suspect that a mother I'm working with is suffering from trauma after giving birth, I continue to ask her questions. For example, what are your complaints? Do you often have night-mares or flashbacks about the birth? Do you experience heart palpitations, stress, anger outbursts, etc? These are some of the symptoms that mothers with birth trauma walk around with. If therapy with me is not enough, I refer these mothers to a good EMDR (eye movement desensitization and reprocessing) thera-pist. EMDR is a psychotherapeutic remedy designed to relieve the distress associated with traumatic memories.[7]

I suffered from birth trauma myself, after the birth of my oldest daughter. I was constantly angry with the entire world and didn't understand why I was feeling that way. When my therapist suggested EMDR, I didn't know if it would help me. In retro-spect, it was the best thing I could have ever done for myself. I can't express how wonderful it felt to be free of all the pain and sadness. I can recommend it to everyone.

But if EMDR isn't for you, I recommend that you keep talking about your birth trauma. Start talking as soon as possible right after the birth, with your partner, a good friend, or anyone you trust or feel comfortable with. But if you feel up to it, try and talk to your midwife or doctor. Tell them that you were left feeling awful after the birth. If there's a way you think they could have handled things differently, tell them. In this way, you get it off your chest and the healthcare professional can (hopefully) learn from your experience.

First time outside after delivery

When you first go outside with your newborn, it can feel like you're running a marathon. A walk around the block can leave you completely exhausted. This is perfectly normal. A friend of mine was overconfident and thought she could handle doing some shopping. She almost collapsed in the store, because she couldn't handle it at all. The pain, the tiredness, the stimuli of the store, and all those people were just too much for her. For your first foray out with your partner and baby, plan just a short trip around the block. If it doesn't work out, you'll soon be home. Most mothers really enjoy that first time outside with their sprout. It can feel wonderful to be introducing your baby to the world, and vice versa, but please build up slowly until you can walk for half an hour without getting completely exhausted.

Letting things go

Some mothers get really anxious once the baby has arrived, feeling as though they have absolutely no control over anything. They want their old life back, which was organized, wellarranged, and well planned. These new mothers yearn for the days when they could go into the city spontaneously, alone or with friends. It can be very painful to leave their old life behind and embrace their new life as a mother. It's important to discuss these feelings.

It doesn't matter who you talk to, but do talk about it! It's completely normal that you have to find your way into your new role. All mothers do.

You can try to maintain the illusion of control for as long as you want. You can indeed go a long way with a routine, and doing that helped me a lot. But there are many other things that you have absolutely no control over. For example, you might set Thursday as your cleaning day. But then your child gets sick and wants to hang on to you like a koala bear. Good luck trying to vacuum. I've completely given up on a neat house. Ask yourself why you care so much that your house is not always in perfect shape. What does it matter if it isn't always super clean?

Learning that you can't be in total control can be a positive life lesson. Be kind to yourself, stop checking everything all the time, and let life come as it comes. 'I accept' is my credo.

Being judged for having a C-section

I don't know why, but having a C-section is often looked down upon. Nowadays, many women opt for natural, nonmedicated home births. Doulas, midwives, and natural birthing coaches are hot and happening.

So when women end up having a C-section after being in labour for days, they can feel as though they've failed. Or when they get a planned Caesarean, they feel a need to explain to the world why they had one. When I gave birth to our second child by C-section, my gynaecologist came up and congratulated me for doing just as amazing a job as any woman who had a natural birth.

It was nice of her to say that. But later I thought that she felt the need to say that and that I needed to hear it didn't make sense. I think every birth is hard, whether you're having a meds-free home birth or a C-section. Having a C-section is not an easy way out. It involves major surgery, and the pain after is no joke. I have had both types of birth and both were intense.

Judging women for having a C-section is ludicrous. Let's all agree on one thing: Giving birth is hard work and we should applaud each other instead of being critical.

Breasts leaking

Another fun thing you can expect when you breastfeed is leaking nipples. You'll need nursing pads inside your bra that will make sure you won't leak through your bra. I've leaked through my bra and top many times—when I was in the gym (thank god everyone thought I was sweating), grocery shopping, in the car, etc. I was pumping a lot, but I had a very high milk production.

Basically, I used nursing pads 24/7. But you probably won't want to wear your nursing bra during sex. I know a lot of nursing mothers who feel embarrassed to take their bras off during sex. I totally understand you. I was like that all the way. And I spilled some serious milk on my husband. My boobs were like the Trevi Fountain in Rome. They kept swinging milk out there, unstoppable. When this happens to you (and it probably will), don't stress about it, okay? It doesn't have to be a passion killer. Just talk to your partner about it, explain what might happen and that it's all normal. And if you don't feel comfortable taking your bra off, leave it on! Put some nursing pads in or wear a nice negligee. Do what feels right for you. Follow your gut feeling, as with all things in life.

Breastfeeding and weight loss

You might hear that breastfeeding ensures that you'll lose weight in no time after childbirth. I hate to disappoint you, but breastfeeding isn't an automatic supersonic fat burner for every mother. It wasn't for me. There are undoubtedly some women out there for whom it was. For those women, feel free to skip this part.

The pounds really don't all of a sudden fly off your hips. There's another important factor at play: hormones. After delivery, your body hangs on to the extra body fat for a while. How long this goes on for varies from person to person. It's nature's way of protecting you and your baby: If food was suddenly scarce, you'd still be able to breastfeed. I actually lost weight when I stopped breastfeeding.

CHAPTER 9

Chat Openly and Honestly with Other Mothers

Rest easy, real mothers.
The very fact that you worry
About being a good mom
Means that you are already one

Throughout this book, I've written about the importance of talking about how you're feeling, and not bottling it up. Talking is incredibly healing, and something that helped me enormously in my recovery, which is why the topic of confiding in others deserves its own chapter.

Of course, not every woman has postpartum depression after giving birth. There are plenty of moms getting on with their lives almost like nothing happened. But the women who had more complicated experiences, be it PPD or not, are likely to understand you the best. Try to find one (or more) of those women, and talk about your thoughts and feelings with her. You'll both find recognition in each other's stories, believe me. And if you don't take the first plunge and open up, who will? Besides, every person I talked to knew a woman who had suffered from postpartum depression, either their mother or their niece or their colleague or their friend. You're not alone.

Postpartum depression is an emotional roller coaster that takes its toll on you as a person and as a mother. It's likely that years later, strong emotions will still arise when you talk about it or even just think about it. I still get choked up by a memory of me walking down the stairway in our old apartment building, having those horrible intrusions and visualizing how I could throw my baby down those stairs. I would *never* do that in real life, of course, but the thoughts were so brutal and vivid. My experience was made even more difficult by not knowing that many mothers went through the same thing. I felt so alone, because I hadn't talked about it. If I had only known then what I know now. One day I met a sweet 60-year-old, Deborah, at a children's birthday party. She regularly babysits her grandchildren. She whispered softly, in a corner of the room, that she had gone through a postpartum depression as well, more than 30 years ago. Deborah hadn't discussed it with anyone at the time. She felt deeply ashamed back then. Only now did she did dare talk openly about it, because she knew that I had experienced the same thing. Her trauma was still present during our conversation. Deborah was afraid of knives when her babies were little, because she was terrified she'd hurt her baby with one. Deep inside, she obviously knew that she would never harm her child, yet the intrusive thoughts kept coming back. To this day, Deborah can't stand to hear crying babies or see knives. I believe that had she been able to talk about her feelings at the time, and get the help she needed, she wouldn't still feel so traumatized. You can avoid long-term trauma by talking about your emotions and doubts with other mothers and with a professional who can help you.

Find a mama guru

Motherhood is sometimes one big puzzle. One way to help yourself figure things out is to find a mama guru—a mother or grandmother with more experience. Start asking her anything you can think of. Questions about the pregnancy, delivery, and the period after that. Your mama guru could be a close friend, your sister, a neighbour, any mother who knows you well and who will be honest with you about everything, and I mean EVERYTHING. Not everyone can find that person, of course. I didn't. But if you don't find your own, please don't worry. I've written this book to fill that role as best I can, and you can find my communities online and communicate with other women who know what you're going through. You can read my blogs under my English instagram: @thisispostpartum or the Frou

Frou Begeleiding Facebook page. I run a Dutch account, where I also blog in English: @geenrozewolk (which means not on cloud nine). You can find me there or through e-mail: info@ froufroubegeleiding.nl. I also do Skype consults worldwide with moms who feel the same way as I did back then. Whatever way works, I'm always here for you.

Fellow companions

A client once said to me, 'I just didn't dare tell anyone because I was ashamed to death of what I thought and felt.' Although that is perfectly understandable, if she had instead just thought *Sod it* and shared her story anyway, she would have heard that many other women go through what she was going through. Knowing this wouldn't have made her problems go away, but it might have made her feel less lonely and given her a sense of solidarity, which is precisely what we all need. Look for a safe environment where you can share your story, a place where you can talk freely without being interrupted and without being judged, a relaxing place where you can be yourself and where you are understood and taken seriously, a place where mothers support each other and there is room for all your thoughts and emotions, a place where no one says, 'You can't say that!'

If you don't talk about your negative feelings and thoughts about motherhood, you'll become increasingly isolated. Sharing your feelings and experiences diminishes your feeling of loneliness, and the more you open up, the more you will find fellow sufferers, other moms who also want nothing more than to be heard and understood.

I believe so strongly in the healing power of talking to like-minded people that I organize group walks in the woods for my clients. Gradually, I see mothers getting better. They flourish, drop their masks, and go home with a sense of relief. You don't have to solve everything all by yourself. It's okay to ask for help or advice. It's okay that you don't do everything perfectly. No one is judging you as harshly as you judge yourself. Find an inner voice that lifts you up instead of bringing you down.

One of the mothers in my walking group said to me, 'I feel like I've stepped into a warm bath.' I was so happy to hear that, because that is why I created the group. I wanted them all to know that they weren't the only mother struggling with motherhood.

Therapy

When I first started talking about feeling depressed after our oldest daughter was born, it felt like an enormous rock was being lifted off my chest, letting me finally breathe. When I first met my therapist, I was too ashamed of my intrusive thoughts to tell her about them. I only told her that I was afraid of something bad happening to my baby because of me. After five sessions, I finally told her about my intrusions. When she told me that many, many mothers experience the same thing, and that she had even had those thoughts, and that the intrusions are simply a warning system in the brain that helps a mother care for her child, I finally got it. I wasn't a bad mom. I was actually a good mom. My brain was just very busy making sure nothing awful was going to happen to my child. Weirdly enough, the terrible thoughts were a good thing. The relief I felt was extraordinary.

My therapist told me about other women's experiences and was open about her own. These true stories gave me hope. I do the same with my clients, and when they ask me personal questions about motherhood, I answer them as honestly as possible. I think talking to a therapist is healing in every aspect of the word. It helps you understand yourself better, but it also offers you a slightly different perspective, so you can find yourself thinking and behaving in new, more helpful, ways.

'I felt so ashamed'

During our trip through America, an American mother who also had postpartum depression told us that she had read all the books and therefore had felt well prepared for motherhood. The prospect of becoming a mother was all positivity. Then she said, 'What no one prepared me for was how incredibly painful and difficult breastfeeding could be. I was in pain all the time.' Not only that, but no one had told her that some women may experience postpartum depression. From her experiences, it seemed like almost no one talks openly about it. She gradually felt more and more isolated, to the point where it was paralyzing. She said, 'I'd given birth to a beautiful baby, a beautiful, healthy girl, and everyone was so happy. Except me. I cried uncontrollably, for hours, and I just couldn't understand why.' She said she didn't understand why she wasn't just happy. Then the fear started. 'How on earth am I going to take care of this little creature for the rest of my life? Can I even do that at all?' And then to top it all off, she started feeling anxious about her relationship with her partner, too. 'I had these visions that my husband would leave me for a nicer, younger version of me and that he'd leave me and the baby. When he came home late, I'd start quizzing him about where he had been, and who with.'

She thought about seeking help but didn't dare take that step. 'I was so ashamed of my thoughts that I didn't want anyone to know what was going on in my head. I didn't want anyone to know that we weren't having the fairy tale postpartum period that everyone always talks about. Because that's what everyone thinks, right? You have a baby and a husband, which means being blissfully happy.' She felt guilty. She was married to her high school sweetheart and the baby was the crowning glory of their happiness and they'd live happily ever after. She also admitted that her reluctance to talk about the problems was a pride issue. It was hard for her to admit that she was struggling. She knew the terrible stories of mothers who did something to their child, so she thought, *I don't have that. I don't want to hurt my child, so it probably isn't postpartum depression, right?* Only after her daughter was six months old did she accept that she was suffering from PPD.

I really felt for my American friend. If only we had met sooner in life, we could have connected and validated each other's experiences. I think that if she'd had more mommy friends or a mama guru, she would have felt less isolated. The postpartum period can be incredibly hard at times, and during those times you just need a shoulder to cry on, someone to listen to you and where you can find some recognition.

Unsolicited advice

When you start to share your story with others, you'll find that some people are less keen on listening and more keen on giving advice…advice that you're not always looking for. No matter how good their intentions, sometimes the advice these people give you is not exactly what you need as a new mother. Try not to take it personally. The other person only wants to help. You can say that you appreciate that they want to help you but what you need right now is someone to listen to you or give you a hug. Or if you want to be even gentler, you could say, 'I know what I need to do, and I'm going to do that. But in the meantime, I'd really love to get this off my chest and let you know how I've been feeling. Do you mind listening?' That's it. Put the advice aside or write it down for when you're ready and if you feel it might be helpful. Otherwise, discard it!

Remember that even the moms who get hailed as a 'relaxed mother' (by themselves or by others) aren't always so relaxed. They also often have their own problems and stress factors that they might choose not to discuss. You don't always know what's going on behind closed doors, so don't compare yourself with them. With my second child Emmi, on the outside I looked like one of those "relaxed moms". Me! Me, who used to triple check whether Livia's swaddle was properly fastened, so she couldn't suffocate in the cloth wrapped around her. I was so scared all the time. But the second time was really different. I felt more secure and didn't have to read everything there was to know about anything. So don't be fooled – those moms who look super relaxed might not always have felt that way.

Dealing with ignorance

Some people may not be able to handle you talking about your thoughts and feelings. This happened to me after I posted my first blog about PPD and it went viral. Several Dutch media outlets picked up on it and it was on one of their Facebook pages. One lady felt the need to post this comment: 'Well, we all have an off day sometimes. It doesn't mean you should hide in your bed or cry all the time. Just put your back into it and move on.' I felt hurt and humiliated by her comment and started to doubt myself. Should I be able to "just move on"? Thoughtless reactions can really hurt, and it sure as hell hurt me. I decided not to read any comments on open Facebook pages again. I felt so vulnerable and that lady obviously didn't have a clue about postpartum depression. Nor did she have any empathy. Back then, I couldn't give a witty response to my online bully. But these days I can, so when someone treats me without respect, I call them on it right away. Set some strong boundaries for yourself, too, and explain to the person in question that you feel very uncomfortable with how they're acting or talking to you.

A client once told me about her deeply unhelpful mom friend who apparently had it all together. My client confided in her about her insecurities and how much she missed her old life. Her friend responded like she was being crazy and ungrateful. 'You wanted a baby, right? So take care of her and don't whine so much.' My client was shocked. She stopped talking about her feelings right then and there. Most people will not be like this, though, far from it. And now that there is more in the media about PPD and a bigger focus on mental health in general, attitudes should continue to improve.

I'd always recommend trying to stay as calm as possible, but look, we're all human and I'm certainly not always calm. My best friend and I once had a huge fight over the phone. We were both a couple of months postpartum, and I don't even remember why we were arguing. But we had very different opinions about the matter, whatever it was. I started screaming, then she started screaming, and at some point my husband ran into our bedroom and pleaded with me to end the conversation. I responded with, 'Oh no, it's all good. She's screaming, too. I think we're getting somewhere.' When I think back to that moment, it makes me laugh. We all laugh about it now. But the bottom line is that we have to have respect for each other's opinions, experiences, and stories. A heated discussion can clear the air, as it did between me and my friend, but being disrespectful or lacking in empathy toward a vulnerable person is an absolute no-go.

How to give advice

Sometimes mothers like to receive advice, usually when they've explicitly asked for it. As I wrote in the mama guru section (page 135), there's a great deal of wisdom to be gained from other people's experiences. But some mothers don't respond well to unsolicited advice. They can misinterpret it as criticism or they feel that people should mind their own business. And I can understand that. There's a lot of unwanted advice-giving in the world of new mothers, and it isn't always pleasant to hear. For example, I had a client with twins. She stopped breastfeeding because it was exhausting her, and she didn't feel as though she had enough milk for both of them, so she switched to formula. Great decision, because it was a huge relief for her and she finally could get some sleep. But some of her friends didn't agree with her decision. They felt the need to judge her, talk back at her, and even send her unsolicited links to websites full of pro breastfeeding propaganda. She felt defeated and that she was being judged by the people she should feel most safe with: her friends, who should have had her back. People she had confided in, told her deepest, darkest secrets to. She never expected them to 'turn on her' as she put it. She felt guilty and shamed by her inner circle. It was heart breaking.

How do you know if someone is open to receiving advice? I think it's a matter of listening to your gut or intuition. If it's a good friend of yours, ask if she wants advice. If a friend is venting about a problem, ask her if she wants to brainstorm solutions with you or if she just wants to vent a bit. Either is fine. If you don't know the mother? Then I'd be careful. Better stay on the safe side. Advice can be well intended, but not every mom wants it.

Keep talking

Processing your postpartum depression involves ups and downs. Talking about it with others will make the process easier because you'll no longer feel so alone. But even if you've been declared depression-free by your therapist, those negative feelings don't just suddenly disappear. They may occasionally reappear and you may find yourself back in that spiral of negative thoughts and feelings. The key here is to talk about it again. Don't be afraid of what others might think or say about you. The only thing you can influence in life is you. You can't control other people's reactions, so focus on yourself and your family. Allow any negative thoughts and feelings to be there, because it's perfectly normal to have them. Acknowledge them and then let them drift away.

Continue to share your insecurities and concerns with others. Whatever happens, keep being as open and communicative as possible. Yes, sometimes you'll feel like people are getting bored: 'There she goes again with all her problems', but be kind to yourself. Don't try to mind read. 'Keep sharing' is the motto, regardless of your own judgmental thoughts. It will really help you progress further through this difficult phase. Crucially, it will also encourage other people to open up and confide in you, too. Together, slowly, we can break down the wall of silence surrounding postpartum depression.

Social media

Social media is a fantastic medium: You can find anything and share everything. On the other hand, there's also a lot of bullying. You can imagine that new mothers, full of worries and anxiety, start looking for some guidance, something to hold on to. They visit various platforms where they find contradictory answers to questions they didn't know they had. Some mothers share their personal experiences online, which can be an outlet for their grey cloud thoughts, but doing that can invite cruel comments from people who don't think how their comments may affect the people reading them. This can be very harmful, making the depression worse and reinforcing the mother's feelings of not being good enough.

The solution is to stop looking at those websites and discuss with your partner, good friend, doctor, or therapist why you're having a hard time. Consider deleting your Facebook account or changing the settings so you don't get annoying notifications. With Instagram, I recommend unfollowing absolutely everyone whose posts make you feel bad about yourself. That supermodel mom who's back on the Victoria's Secret catwalk one month after giving birth? That mom friend showing off about how her baby sleeps through the night two weeks post-partum? Only follow accounts that offer support, humour, or somehow make you feel better. I also recommend following these hastags: #thisismotherhood #notsomumsy #momcom-munity #keepitreal.

It takes a village

The saying is that takes a village to raise a child, but we don't have that village anymore. Our parents might work or live far away. Our relatives have busy lives and might live in another state or even a different country. Your friends might have fami-lies themselves and are busy combining work and motherhood. Because of this, I argue that it's even more important to find a close parent community where everyone can help each other out more. For example, finding other moms in your neigh-bourhood and starting a babysitting rota. Or everyone cooks an extra plate and takes it to the overwhelmed woman who can barely take care of herself and the baby, so she can fill her freezer. You could also start an online Facebook group where you can connect, share your stories, and ask questions. Let's build the village ourselves! Let's create a safety net for all new mothers.

Of course, you don't have to share your feelings and thoughts nonstop if you don't want to. For example, if you're having a nice lunch with a friend and you're talking about her vaca-tion plans, you really don't have to change the subject abruptly and start talking about your depression. Do what feels right at that moment. Just remember that wherever you are, there is a mother out there who totally gets you and who you can always contact through the magic of social media, if you need to. Including yours truly.

CHAPTER 10

Taking Your Child to Day Care

*Real mothers aren't perfect
And perfect mothers aren't real*

Motherhood is hard work and we all need to take a break from it every once in a while. This is completely normal; in fact, I think breaks are absolutely essential. The next time you yearn for some time to yourself, ask your partner (if you have one) to take over for a bit, or call a friend, neighbour, or mother- or father-in-law. Whomever. From time to time, you'll really need to recharge, and everyone will understand, because a happy mom makes for a happy baby. One of my mom friends once told me that whenever she got home stressed from work, her children were always grumpy, so she decided to flick the switch and come home in a good mood. She noticed that they became happier and more relaxed, too. "So now I restart the day when I come home from work and pick up the kids from daycare. It is a new phase of the day with new energy and that works like a charm."

Sometimes, I feel overwhelmed after a day of work and then being with my kids. My work as a therapist is amazing; it doesn't even feel like work, to be honest. But of course, it's also intense. I'm not only seeing clients but writing new material, blogs, etc., as well as training maternity nurses on early recognition of PPD. My mind is all over the place. You can imagine that I need to unwind after a day of work, but I have to rush to the childminder to pick up my kids, who may well be tired and grouchy, too. I needed to figure out a way to calm my system before I got there.

I decided to start walking to the childminder and to do a walking meditation exercise en route. I breathe in slowly and exhale consciously. I let go of any negative thoughts I might have, because my older daughter in particular will pick up on them. Once I arrive at the childminder's house, I cheerlead myself: *I'm a good mother, I can pull this off.* And only once I've said that do I ring the doorbell. If I feel like I'm still not ready, I take another walk around the block. It's made such a difference. I no longer arrive stressed out, and it means I can also handle my kids' tantrums at the end of the day much better. They're tired, too, and they want their mama, so I need to be ready for that. Once I started the walking meditation, I felt so much more confident that I could handle the evening ritual by myself (which I often have to, because my husband is away a lot).

Full disclosure: Even though I'm a big advocate of it now, it took me a while to take my first daughter to day care. I just couldn't at first. I also decided to hire a babysitter who could help me out between 5 and 7:30 in the evening. Our babysitter, a young girl who's in college and the daughter of a good friend of mine, helps me feed the kids and put them to bed. Not only does she provide an extra set of hands, she also really helps with Emmi's tantrums. She lightens the mood in the house and I love that. When we've finished eating, she reads them a book or watches TV with them while I unload the dishwasher, clean up the kitchen, and fold some laundry. At bedtime, she puts one of the girls to bed while I do the bedtime ritual with the other one. I don't feel stressed or exhausted, because I know there's someone who can help me out until both girls are asleep.

There are people out there who think that a mother that needs help with dinner and bedtime isn't able to cope with motherhood. I say, they can roll their eyes at me all they want. I learned the hard way what happens if you don't ask for help. I know when I need help and I'm not afraid to ask for it. Period.

One of my clients told me, 'It was all too much for me. Sometimes I dreamt that I'd jump on a plane and leave. I was desperate to be alone and to not have any demands on my time.' You can't jump on a plane on a whim, but fortunately, you can leave your child with a babysitter for an afternoon. Taking your child to someone who will take care of him doesn't make you a bad mom; it can be a lifesaver and is sometimes the very best thing to do.

How to trust someone else with your child

How hard is it to admit that you don't really trust anyone with your child except your partner? (And even then…) For many mothers, taking their child to a day care centre or leaving him with a childminder or nanny is a big deal. They don't trust a stranger with their child. This fear can be overwhelming and trap you in a negative cycle. The more you worry, the more you could benefit from some baby-free time, but the more you think about leaving your baby with someone else, the more you worry… For me, it was impossible to leave my child with a complete stranger, even when that stranger was a highly educated childcare professional. I longed for some alone time, but I just couldn't do it. I got crankier and crankier and at some point my husband said, 'That's it. You need to do something now, because you're been stuck in this negative cycle for ages and nothing is happening. You need to take Liv to a nanny or day care.' I knew he was right, but of course I threw a fit, because I was terrified. After I calmed down, I remembered what my therapist had said to me: that I needed more time for myself, at least one day a week alone. I took a look at the nearest day care centre in our neighbourhood. I could barely keep it together, I felt so much anxiety. Once I started talking to some of the staff, I started crying. I explained my situation between tears and fears. The lady was so kind and understanding. The week after, Liv did her trial, as they called it.

After that, every week I had an entire day to myself. At first, I slept, but after a few weeks I started to work out, go shopping, or have lunch with a friend. I loved every minute of my time off. Of course, I called the centre regularly to check how Liv was doing, but she did great. It was one of the best decisions I could have ever made, and it really helped me recover from my PPD.

Once you've tasted freedom again, you'll realize how much you missed it. And once you've seen how well day care can work, you'll feel progressively more confident and relaxed dropping your baby off for the day. You'll find yourself coming out of the downward cycle. Admitting to yourself that you actually don't trust anyone with your child is already a big step. The next step is to discuss your fears with your partner or a good friend, either of whom can be a rational sounding board.

Start thinking about childcare early on

You have several options when it comes to the care of your child, and you don't always have to rely on a nanny or day care. I know childcare is expensive; this weighed heavily on my mind. I had lost my job while pregnant, so I was home without any pay. But I asked around in my inner circle if anyone wanted to babysit and was surprised by how many people were willing to give up some of their free time to babysit Liv.

It's important to start thinking early on, even as early as during your pregnancy, about what kind of childcare you'd prefer. Discuss the options with your partner. This is important because if you suffer from postpartum depression after giving birth, your partner can remind you of what you talked about, even if by then you feel you just can't face anything. Another reason for early discussion is that childminders are often fully booked in advance.

Here are a few things you might want to consider:

- Do you want a day care centre with several groups?
- Do you want something on a smaller scale, such as a babysitter or nanny?
- Do you want someone you know, such as a grandfather and grandmother, to come and look after your child in your own home?

My own experience

Tim was working long hours and so I was home all day with Liv. My psychologist kept telling me that it was very important that I also made time for myself. Apparently a quick tea break while the baby is napping doesn't count! No, what we're talking about here are genuine, blissful, relaxing hours all for yourself, where you can do whatever you want, from catching up with a friend to getting your hair cut. Problem was, I didn't feel like doing that at all, at first.

When Liv was four months old, a friend finally persuaded me to drop Liv off at day care. She came with me for moral support. We'd have lunch together, then I'd pick Liv up two hours later. Simple. Right. It caused a paralyzing, almost suffocating fear. I lost count of the number of times I told Tim that I couldn't do it, couldn't cope. When it was finally time for me to drop my girl off, my emotions were overwhelming. I kept a brave face for my child, said goodbye to her with a thousand kisses, then walked straight out of the centre, swallowing my tears. Once outside,

I cried until I couldn't cry any more. I'd done it, the one thing I thought I could never do: I'd left my baby with a complete stranger. My girlfriend assured me that it would get easier, that Liv was going to love it at day care and that once I saw that, I wouldn't feel so bad. She was right, of course, but it didn't feel that way at the time.

We had lunch at a restaurant nearby and enjoyed a cup of tea in the sun. After an hour I called the day care centre to check how Liv was doing. My girl was happily fast asleep. I hung up the phone and sighed with relief. Picking her up was a party! As soon as I walked into the room, she immediately turned toward me, making high squeaky sounds and reaching out her arms toward me. At that moment I was filled with joy and pride. I was so proud that I had managed to endure leaving her. So proud of her for doing so well. So proud that I'd broken the negative spiral. And so proud because I knew that from that day on I'd have time for myself every week.

Liv and I gradually progressed from a few hours to a whole day. The first time I had a whole day alone at home without a baby was intense. Of course I felt guilty (when did I not feel guilty?), but I got quickly used to occasionally being without my daughter. In the morning after I had taken her to day care, I would exercise. It was a nice way of grounding myself and releasing some pent-up energy. It still is. Then I would try and do something social. It's so important to catch up with friends (particularly friends who don't have children) and it isn't an expensive activity.

Top tips for coping with daycare

- Make sure you find a nanny or day care that you feel comfortable with. Listen to your intuition.
- Stick with your decision, even if you rethink it after giving birth and start thinking that you won't do it.
- Share your fears about leaving your baby with a stranger.
- Ask your partner to take your child (or go together).
- If you can't ask a partner, ask a good friend to help you.
- Agree with the babysitter or nanny that you can call after an hour to check in on your baby.
- Ask them to send you a photo of your child.
- Tell them you're going to call often during the day, because you feel anxious.

Finding yourself again

Recovery from depression cannot be rushed. It is what it is: a depression. Nobody truly understands what you're going through unless they themselves have also gone through it. And even then, everyone's experience is different. Don't feel as though you have to rush your recovery, but please don't let your fears constantly pull you back, either. Allow yourself to occasionally dream about how you want to organize your life in the long run. What do you want to do the most in this world? No, I'm not saying that every person with depression must change their lives drastically. But try to think about what makes you really happy. This could be a long-discarded hobby, or a long-held dream of travelling. Maybe in this present moment, it's the last thing you want to think about, but one day you'll feel better again and you'll be ready.

I found it very helpful to dream about how nice my life could be with my baby. Before having a baby, my daydreams mostly didn't include a baby. For many mothers, the postpartum period is almost like a mourning process. They often recall memories of pre-motherhood, from trips they took, to summer festivals spent drinking and partying until the sun went down (or came up). It can be hard to lose your old identity.

Once you've become a mother, taking some alone time can help you rediscover your identity. What did you do before you had kids? Maybe you liked yoga: Please do that again. Or maybe you devoured books: Go dive deep into a book that has nothing to do with raising a child. Reconnecting with your old self is important, because besides being a mother (which is huge) you also need to do fun stuff for you, to remember who you were and to love that side of yourself again.

Being a relaxed mother

Being a chill mom is a bit of a holy grail. My friends and I used to talk jealously about so-and-so who was just so relaxed. So, as well as being a perfect mother, we also have to make it look really easy... I felt as though I needed to achieve that relaxed state in order to be a successful mom. The words would echo in my head: *You have to be relaxed. Don't be so stressed out all the time.* But when I finally became a mother, I was anything but relaxed.

As a mother you go through different phases, just as your child does. In some situations, you'll be flexible and relaxed, but there will be many situations where you're not. For example, when your child is behaving appallingly, you might wonder what crawled into him. *Do we need an exorcism right now?* I often asked myself when I looked at my toddler. Do what your mother's heart tells you to do, and if that means calling the doctor every week with a new ailment, so be it.

Don't stress yourself out trying to be the perfect relaxed mom. Just trust that you'll become more relaxed as time goes on because you'll get to know your child and the signals he's giving you better and better. And on top of that, you'll grow in confidence in yourself and your new role as a mother, and you won't feel as insecure.

Finding a new balance

Finding the balance between going back to work (or following further education) and taking care of your little one calls for a new balance in your life. You'll probably find it difficult in the beginning, although not all parents do. What works for a lot of mothers is a lot of advance prepping. So, for example, hang your work outfit ready to go in your closet, pack your work bag the night before, shower at night so you don't have to get up crazy early in the morning, etc. What I really liked was getting myself ready and only then getting my baby out of bed, so I didn't have to stress about her while I was getting ready. You'll soon find a routine that works for you, and the more preparations you can do the night before, the easier your mornings will be.

Once you're back at work or in college, expect to be thinking about your baby a lot in the beginning. It's perfectly normal. Allow yourself to call the nanny or day care to check up on him, and scroll through pictures of him during lunchtime. All moms do, trust me! Sometimes you might have to leave early because he's sick, or you might need to skip a meeting in order to be on time for pick-up. All moms find this stressful, so be as kind to yourself as possible. Don't judge yourself for not working as late as you used to or for not going out on a drinking bender with your colleagues on a Friday night. You have different priorities now. Do what feels right for you and stick with that. There's no right way, so do it your way.

I studied mostly when Liv was in day care. I used a lot of the time to read and do homework. Studying helped me sharpen my brain again after the pregnancy fog had lifted. I took Liv to day care at 9 a.m. and picked her up at 5 p.m. or before. She was always so happy to see me and of course I loved seeing her little face again. Once I got used to her going to day care, I didn't find going back to studying hard. Because I found the early days of motherhood so stressful, anything that came after was peanuts. I did miss Liv sometimes, but I also enjoyed my study days and made the most of them. I also found that I began to really cherish when Liv and I did have the whole day together. I appreciated those moments so much more than when Liv and I were together absolutely all the time. A change of food makes you want to eat, my grandmother always said, and that makes sense, if you ask me.

Nowadays, when the girls are in school and nursery, I'm usually at work. But on the occasional day where I'm home alone, I do a little dance. I'm home. Alone. Without anyone asking me for anything. I can drink a cup of tea without it getting cold. I can switch on blasting music and dance through the living room. I can binge watch my new favourite Netflix series. Yes, I also work on those days. But I always take some time for myself.

CHAPTER 11

The Importance of Self-Care

Just wing it!
Life,
Eyeliner.
Everything.

Before my first baby, I was the Carrie type from *Sex and the City*, always in heels, outfits, and flawless makeup. I really enjoyed rummaging through vintage shops and markets to score that one perfect item. It was a lot of fun and a playful, creative experience for me. Clothes were a way of expressing myself. My husband didn't get it. He says the vintage stores smell funny. So I used to go by myself and have a blast. I still do, actually. It's one of my favourite things to do. In Utrecht, where we used to live, there are wonderful vintage stores. I also loved to stroll down car boot sales or vintage markets. I loved to dress up and play around with clothes, jewellery, shoes, and bags. I still do, but with two kids it can be a challenge. All the same, I still like to think of myself as the Dutch Carrie.

But I didn't care about any of that during those first weeks postpartum. Having fun was the furthest thing from my mind. I wore sweatpants and a baseball shirt. The shirt was chosen because it had buttons on the front, which made it easy to breast-feed. 'Nice and easy' quickly became my philosophy. Add a messy topknot on my head (instead of styled curls), zero makeup, and my slippers and you have my new-mom look perfectly nailed. Of course it's totally okay if you spend less time on your appearance than I do. We don't have to look like those Insta-perfect moms, right? For some women, it might be a welcome relief to not worry so much about appearances, but not paying any attention whatsoever can be a sign that you're neglecting yourself in other ways, too, and this can keep the depression cycle going for longer. No, spending time in nature alone, treating yourself to a delicious latte, or getting a haircut or a massage isn't going to cure the depression. But with time, these little pleasurable treats you can give yourself accumulate. You learn to enjoy things again, and more importantly, you learn to treat yourself with care and attention.

I know first-hand that it can be incredibly hard to do nice things for yourself—in a depression we stop enjoying anything—but actually it does really, really help, because you trick your brain into thinking you're worth that latte or new lipstick or well-deserved rest.

How I learnt to be nicer to myself

When I started to find space in my head to try new things again, I didn't know where to start. I'd completely lost myself and didn't know who I was anymore. Being nicer to myself was the best advice I got from my therapist. I literally had to ask myself: *What did I used to do when I had time off? What did I like? Where did I want to go?* I talked to Tim about my therapist telling me that I needed more time for myself, so when he was home on the weekends, I'd meet up with a friend or go to the gym. Having lunch somewhere or working out were some of my favourite things to do before kids. At first I felt guilty, of course. (We've already established that when you become a mother, guilt and shame sit on your shoulders, yip-yapping in your ears all day. I would love to flick them off my shoulders.) I also tried on new clothes, two sizes bigger. I felt like I needed to let go of my old size. Maybe I'd fit into those old skinnies again, or maybe not. Both were okay. So I'd wash and curl my hair, put on a new or reinvented outfit, and head out the door. It felt so liberating. Obviously, the curls were a lot of effort and just for fun, or for a special occasion. That messy bun—a high topknot—never left, by the way. People call it my signature look now. I'm fully embracing it. I think the bun is a mother's version of a crown. Sometimes I wear mine with a leopard print scrunchie.

I've tried to incorporate more self-care activities into my daily life. Even the smallest things can really help. I've noticed that if I take care of myself inside and out, I feel so much better. In this hectic life, it's important to really learn how to put yourself first sometimes. Yes, of course there is guilt involved, because when don't we experience that? But you deserve to treat yourself every once in a while. I love to go out for a walk, for example. Sometimes I walk through my neighbourhood, but I also love to walk in the woods near my house. This is also where I organize the mom groups. We walk in a group through the forest. We do a walking meditation and then talk about all things postpartum. We also laugh a lot, because I think a good sense of humour about things can really help the situation you're in. Moms feel so much better after this and I enjoy it a lot myself. I also love to get a massage or mani/pedi. It's such a treat that I feel like a different person after. Swimming is also something I really enjoy. Not because I want to lose weight but because I feel very calm and relaxed in the water. Sometimes I swim laps, and sometimes I sit in the jacuzzi. I always come home with rosy cheeks and in a much better mood.

Accumulate positive emotions

Self-care is also about creating positive thoughts and emotions about yourself, life, motherhood, your kids, and more. If you've been having a lot of negative thoughts about motherhood and you can't seem to shake them, please try the exercises in chapter 5 and then say some positive phrases to yourself. The positive affirmations might feel really strange at first, but keep going! Like this: *I love myself unconditionally. I accept myself for who I am. I love myself inside and out. I am valuable. I matter.* You can write these affirmations down and put them all around your house where you'll see them, on the fridge, for example, or on a mirror. I firmly believe that once you start saying these positive things to yourself, even if you don't believe them yet, your heart will eventually follow and you'll start to feel more confident and more loving toward yourself. It's like planting seeds. Positive seeds.

Another nice thing you can do to take care of yourself is keep hand towels infused with your favourite aromatherapy oil in your freezer. You can grab one and place it around your neck or on your forehead after your child has had a tantrum or has just bitten your nipple. Basically, whenever you want to scream. Instead of screaming, try a towel; it makes you feel slightly better!

{ SELF-CARE ROUTINES MY FRIENDS AND I HAVE FOUND HELPFUL }

- Wearing really cozy soft slippers and blankets during the winter months
- Watching nature documentaries
- Using aromatherapy oils and diffusers, especially when we have to do some chore or admin we don't want to do
- Listening to a mindfulness app and meditating in the middle of the day

- Doing a meditation in the woods or when you're going to pick your kids up from day care
- Making hot chocolate for yourself and drinking it before it gets cold (personal fave)

Relationship between inside and outside

Beautician Tamara de Stigter says, ' I often meet young mothers in our salon. These moms have two things in common afterwards: They feel relaxed and they feel more feminine.' During a massage your body produces endorphins and you're likely to end up feeling a little happier and rejuvenated, so if you can, try to schedule one regularly.

Taking care of your appearance isn't about how you look to other people, because who cares about that? It's about how you can make yourself feel. Many women I know are scared of what other people might think of them. I used to be one of those women. I used to go out of the house in full glam mode. My husband taught me how to not care what the world thought of me. I'm so grateful for that. I started to go to the gym, for example, without first doing my hair (hello messy bun). I'd stretch that to days when I didn't have to work and then during holidays abroad where I don't wear any makeup at all. I feel like my skin gets a lot of much-needed rest and a little tan, despite the fact I put at least SPF50 on it. I realized two things: (1) it only matters to you if you're wearing makeup or your best outfit, and (2) strangers don't know how you normally look like, so they'll take you as you are. Why shouldn't you accept and love yourself just the way you are? You deserve it, so please be a little nicer to yourself and shut that inner critic up.

A facial or massage can boost your mood and self-esteem. It can be a revelation to pay yourself just a bit of attention, to remember that you deserve being looked after, too. Do whatever makes you feel good.

Don't go on a shopping spree

I ordered so many clothes when Livia was first born. I think it was because I felt so lost in my postpartum body, I was looking for the new me and thought new clothes would solve that issue. (Ha!) I didn't have a lot of confidence back then, and I think the shopping gave me a feeling of being in control again. Now, after two babies, I know that it isn't about having control, and it doesn't matter how you look on the outside but it does matter how you feel on the inside. I shopped so much that I got to know our delivery guy well. As a matter of fact, I got to know him so well I knew the names of his mom, his dad, his sisters, and his girlfriend. I would even be anxiously asking after his sister once she got to her due date. I shopped till I dropped, and I barely wore half the clothes I ordered. Such a waste of time and money. I could have spent that time on a nap, which I needed much more, or investing in my friendships by checking up on a friend's job interview, or watching some Netflix when my baby was sleeping.

After childbirth it's easy to panic and start spending a great deal of money in an attempt to buy happiness or make ourselves feel more like our old selves again. However, I don't recommend buying an entirely new wardrobe right after childbirth because your shape will change over the next year. Having a few staple outfits that you love and that fit you well as you are now is key.

You don't need a huge number. See which of your favourite tops, leggings, tunics, and dresses you can combine to make a few cute sets. Then hang those sets together in your closet. You can switch it up: On Monday you'll wear it with a blazer on top and on Tuesday with a nice scarf or necklace. This way you won't have to wear the same items every day and you won't get frustrated by not being able to fit into your old wardrobe yet. Plus, think of the convenience of just grabbing an outfit without having to try to put an outfit together during the morning rush hour, because who's in the mood for thinking about accessorizing when the baby is crying and there's been no time for coffee?

Are you kidding me?

Maybe you're feeling so depressed that self-care is absolutely the last thing you want to think about. Perhaps you feel guilty about even doing anything like self-care, because you feel as though you need to spend all your time and energy on your baby or doing chores around the house. You're not alone! I felt like that, too. When I finally decided to go to a hairdresser, I felt immensely guilty about leaving my child to go do something that 'selfish'. But when I came home, I felt like a different person. A fresh haircut and a blow dry can do a lot for you. If you feel like you're not up for any of this, start small. Try to schedule one activity a day that will make you feel better. Go outside. Spend some time walking and breathing fresh air. Feel the wind through your hair, sunlight on your face. Try to be in the present while doing it. It doesn't have to take long. Self-care is also about listening to your body and when it has had enough. When you're ready, expand your self-care to the next level. Maybe visit a friend you haven't seen for a while. Or invite that friend over and go somewhere together. Leaving my baby behind with Tim's mother for the first time wasn't easy for me, but I knew she'd take good care of her, and by the time my hairdresser got all the foils in my hair, I had only texted my mother-in-law once and Liv was fast asleep. I was so proud of Liv, and of myself. I felt relieved and could enjoy sipping my warm tea. That was a major eye opener: I could do something nice for myself and the world didn't come tumbling down.

If all else fails, take a bath! Nutrition and sports coach Nadine de Goed says, 'Happiness can be found in the tiniest things. Just an hour alone in the bathroom with the door closed in a wonderfully warm bath can give you a little boost. A beautiful piece of music and a lovely smelling shower gel helps, too.' You know yourself best, so do what's right for you, find what works for you. Maybe a bath works a treat. Maybe you hate baths, but taking five minutes to look at the birds on your birdfeeder really lifts your mood.

My advice for all new parents is to choose your own path and walk it with confidence. There will be many people who will give you unwanted advice, who will make you feel insecure as a parent, or who will induce anxiety. The thing is, life throws you curveballs, so you need to learn how to handle them. If you decide on a conscious level that you want to believe in yourself, find yourself worthy as a human being and as a mother, something will change inside you. A positive swing will take place. Do the positive affirmations, find the time for self-care as much as you can, and start being incredibly nice to yourself. Then watch the unconditional love for yourself start to grow.

CHAPTER 12

How Your Relationships Can Change

A perfect relationship
Isn't ever actually perfect,
It's just one where both
People never give up

Many couples struggle after their baby is born. Sometimes you lose yourself as a person, but you can also lose sight of each other. I remember one time when Livia was a couple of weeks old. Tim and I had planned to cook a meal together, but one of us fell asleep on the couch. (It wasn't me.) Liv was also napping and I felt p*ssed off that I was the one cooking. Again. I did my best to follow the recipe, but I was exhausted and not thinking straight, so I added salt at least once too many times (okay, probably five times). I also let the meat burn and my husband is a huge meat lover. At some point I started crying and that woke him up. I was shouting that I had ruined "his" meat (I was going to eat it, too, but I completely forgot about that) and then I started yelling that it wouldn't have happened if he hadn't fallen asleep and had been there to help me. Needless to say, the atmosphere in the Timmers household was frosty. We ended up ordering takeout and ate it in silence.

From honeymoon stage to...

If you have a partner, what was your relationship like before you were pregnant? Were you guys lovey dovey? Did you enjoy going to festivals with friends? Did you live at the pub? And what is it like now, post baby? Back in 2005, before Livia was even a twinkle in my eye, Tim and I were madly in love. We met in a club in Utrecht and hit it off right away. Tim was just back from his internship in Johannesburg and I was in college. We both had busy lives, but we always made time for each other. We had our ups and downs and sometimes it was incredibly hard because of his intense work schedule. At some point Tim was doing a PhD plus working over 70 hours a week. Needless to say, we barely saw each other even though we lived together; I sometimes felt neglected and worried about our future together. We argued more when we didn't see each other that much, but we would do a lot of fun stuff together such as trips to Prague, Berlin, and Copenhagen. In the summer we'd go to the beach with a truck full of food and watch the sunset together (I've always been a sucker for sunsets). On good days we felt we had the world at our feet, and we went everywhere we wanted to go—out with friends or to big dance parties. We lived, we laughed, we loved.

After six years, Tim asked me to marry him. We were on an amazing road trip through Botswana, Mozambique, and Zambia. Tim carried my engagement ring with him for weeks, waiting for the right spot to propose. The idea of him carrying that ring everywhere we went, scouting for the perfect romantic location, still fills me with so much love. We were at the Victoria Falls in Zambia, the most beautiful place I've ever been to. He asked a couple of passers-by if they could film us. Tim said to the guy, "Listen, whatever happens, just keep filming." I was like, *what is he doing?* I was just enjoying the incredible view on the waterfalls and its everlasting rainbow. Tim came up to me and started to scramble words. He was clearly nervous. He eventually said, "I love you so much and we've been through a lot. I see my future with you and want to spend the rest of my life with you." With his hat on backward and his backpack still on, he went down on one knee and asked me if I would marry him. I started to laugh, cry, giggle, and yelled, "YESSSSS!!!" We have a photo of that moment; it stands in a prominent spot in our living room. I will cherish that memory forever.

That was then.

Fast forward to 2014. In the throes of PPD, I felt like I was in the deepest sinkhole imaginable. I felt a million miles away from the carefree Tilda who loved travelling with her boyfriend. Tim and I were barely talking. We were exhausted. There was little affection, barely any form of communication, and I felt so lonely. What happened to us?

Who were we before we became parents?

I didn't feel like myself at all right after I had Livia, but deep down, I was still the same Tilda. I just had to find her again. It took a while before I rediscovered myself. My therapist gave me homework assignments, one of which was to spend more time on myself. That meant leaving the house and doing something that didn't have anything to do with my baby or the household. I had to ask myself, *If you had one thing you really wanted to do, what would that be?* I'd always loved shopping, so I decided to stroll through the vintage stores in my city. On a Thursday morning, when the city was still quiet, I walked through the city. I tried on some cute outfits. I bought a nice belt. I met up with a friend for coffee and was home three hours later. I felt a little lighter. What had just happened? I'd finally had a bit of fun.

Friends are often a big part of our identity, especially when we're younger. I think once you've become a mother, it's important to realize you might neglect some of your friends, especially the friends without children. You might justify your neglect by telling yourself that they 'don't get you' or that they 'don't understand what you're going through'. But you could be wrong about that. And more importantly, you probably need your friends now more than ever. Please call your BFF that you haven't seen in weeks or maybe months. Talk to him or her and tell them what you need. You might be surprised by the help they offer, and just talking to them will probably make you feel a lot better, less isolated. Once you actually meet up with them again, it'll be hard not to find some parts of it fun. It's such a change from sitting home with your baby. Relationships can change, not only when you become a mom, but in general. Is that a bad thing? No! Nurture the relationships you have with people who give you energy, and keep people who drain you at a distance. It sounds harsh, but you only have so much energy to give. You'd probably rather save your energy for your partner, your baby, and the friends who are there for you.

After Emmi was born, I had a milder version of the identity crisis I had with Liv. It was easier that time, because I had a new purpose. I had to make sure we got out of the house at 8.00 a.m. so Livia got to school on time. That was a challenge. I showered either crazy early in the morning or late in the evening. In between, there was never any time. I remember asking for help more often, for instance, asking other parents at school if they could drop Liv off on their way home if Emmi was napping or I was feeding her and couldn't leave the house. I felt like Tilda, but a newer, improved version. After all the soul searching I'd done after having Liv, I finally knew who I was. Tilda 2.0. And I liked her right away.

So how do you find yourself again after becoming a mother? I think staying true to yourself is very important. Don't compare yourself to other moms. Don't try to be a 'relaxed mom' if you're the anxious type, like me. I think it's best to take baby steps. Start looking for proof that you're still the person you used to be, instead of thinking about how you've lost yourself. It's normal to lose yourself after giving birth, but it's also common to find yourself again. Go for the 2.0 version of you and start embracing her. Rediscover the things you love and do more of them. Start a relationship with yourself. The best relationship with yourself. That's the most important relationship in your life because it affects every one of your other relationships. You matter! So much. And from the moment you start to see that, you'll never want to let that positive and empowering feeling go.

Getting out of a relationship rut

It happens to almost all couples. You're both so busy with the baby and everything life is throwing at you that you forget to make time for each other. Then night falls and if you're lucky you can chill on the couch and watch Netflix. You barely talk because you're both exhausted, and your main aim is to get to bed as early as possible. The next day is a replica of the day before and it can go on for weeks and months, like *Groundhog Day*. I was a real party girl before I became a mother, going out drinking and dancing until six in the morning, watching the sun rise while biking back home. Now, the wildest thing I do is fall asleep on the sofa instead of the bed. Motherhood was an adjustment, to put it mildly.

But getting permanently stuck in a rut is something you can prevent, I'm convinced. The best way for Tim and me was to spend time together away from the baby. Of course, leaving the baby can be challenging and you may well shed serious tears when you say goodbye to her. I did. I sometimes still do cry when I say goodbye to my babies. More on this shortly. The time you spend together as a couple will help you reconnect in your relationship and also reconnect to your old self. The realization will come that you're not just a mother but a person in your own right.

After the fog of the maternity weeks has cleared up, ask yourself what you normally did on Friday or Saturday night. Did you love hanging out in your local? Then go out and have a beer with your partner in your favourite pub. Did you have a lovely dinner to celebrate a special occasion? Go back to that cosy restaurant and laugh about how much has changed in your lives since you were last there. Come up with something that reminds you of who you were before giving birth. You don't have to swing from the chandeliers until three in the morning; you can just pop out somewhere nearby and go home two hours later if you fancy it. It might feel like an unnecessary ordeal—organizing childcare, worrying about the baby—but investing in your relationship will always be worth it.

The first time out without your baby

What with my PPD, it was particularly hard for me to let a complete stranger babysit. The first time Tim and I went out for dinner was about eight weeks after Liv was born. We were in a rut, and we realized we needed to spend some time together. I chose to ask some friends to watch Liv and they were sweet enough to come over and babysit. That saved me a lot of time and energy looking for a babysitter. Although I would trust these friends with my life, I still found it very hard to leave my baby behind.

I remember that first time we went out to dinner together vividly. My anxiety was acute, but I also knew Tim and I desperately needed some time together, just the two of us. Our relationship needed to be watered, like a plant. Beforehand, I tried to do some meditation and breathing exercises and push through the anxious thoughts I had. I started to get ready, doing my hair, choosing an outfit and shoes and doing my makeup. What was that? Yes, I felt a spark of joy while getting ready. It felt good to pay attention to myself and my marriage again.

When we left the house, I had a lump in my throat. I felt incredibly guilty leaving Liv behind. (Note: She was sound asleep.) I felt guilty because we were going off without her and 'being selfish'. Brushing away my tears, we cycled into Utrecht. Once we arrived at the restaurant I started to calm down. There were so many distractions and I was enjoying my glass of cava. I'd calculated that I could drink exactly one glass of bubbles between pumping without the alcohol getting into my breast milk. We ordered our food and put our phones on the table. Yes, all mothers do that in the beginning. Don't feel guilty or embarrassed about it, it's very normal. After a few months I finally got the confidence to put my phone in my purse on date nights. (Note: My husband still leaves his within reach.) We thoroughly enjoyed our food, which for once did not get cold. We talked about us as a couple, about how we felt about being parents, about our fears and dreams, about things that concerned us. We reconnected and I felt closer to him. I remember falling asleep that night with a lighter feeling in my head and limbs because I knew we were on a positive path again.

After our second baby was born, my relationship with Tim didn't suffer as much. I started to plan date nights sooner, and we still do them regularly. I didn't want a repeat situation of what had happened the first time round, so I looked for a babysitter soon after Emmi was born and found one close to home. Or I asked my parents or friends to watch our girls. The second time was definitely less difficult than the first time. Was it easy? To leave the girls behind, sure. But arranging quality time together can still be a challenge. As I said before, a good relationship is hard work. You can't make a marriage work just overnight. You have to work at it. And having time to communicate with each other and reconnect on a regular basis is invaluable.

I had a client who took her baby to her parents every weekend because she just couldn't take the sleep deprivation anymore. Then she and her partner got to spend time together and actually get some sleep. I thought it was fantastic that she was listening to her body and mind and following her intuition. Of course, she also felt very guilty. I so wish I could magic the guilt away. It's pointless and unhelpful.

Quality time together on a budget

Date nights don't need to be expensive. You don't even need to leave your house. Thank god for Pinterest, where I found some fun ideas for a date night at home. I happen to enjoy cooking, so I took pleasure looking into recipes that are just that little bit more special. But if you don't like cooking, please don't add this as another burden on your to-do list! If your partner is more of a cook, maybe he or she could make you your favourite meal while you put the baby to bed. Or you can ask a friend to help out. I'm not much of a chef (or housewife), to be honest, so I mostly cook simple meals. And when I don't feel like doing that, because I'm exhausted from my day, I just order takeout. It's all good, as long as you feel comfortable with it.

To avoid babysitting costs, perhaps you could ask a favour from your parents or in-laws and suggest a sleepover for your baby at their house. Then you can sleep late the next morning without worrying about the baby waking up. But the simplest option is to let your baby sleep comfortably at home. A date doesn't even have to be in the evening. Sometimes it's logistically easier to have a friend or sibling look after your baby for a few hours one weekend afternoon. You and your partner could do something as simple as going for a walk. The important thing is that you get to talk to each other, to have the kinds of conversation that are impossible to have in snatched minutes between feeds.

Stop multitasking!

Have you ever tried to have an important conversation with a friend who keeps checking their phone? It's unnerving. Even if they're listening, it feels like they're not that interested in what you're saying. So many of us run on autopilot. You run the household, feed the baby, sleep for a few hours, maybe have a quick chat with your partner while washing bottles or checking your phone. Real communication involves speaking about your lived experience, listening carefully to each other, hearing what the other person has to say. One of my clients hit a rough patch in her marriage. Her partner wouldn't do anything to help out with the household, taking care of the kids, doing groceries, etc. They had huge fights about it and were talking about a divorce. When they came to my practice together, I asked them, "What do you want out of this relationship?" They looked at me with foggy eyes; they just didn't know anymore. I suggested they start talking. Just talk.

About anything. The weather, something funny that happened, etc. Anything to get the relationship juices flowing.

Once you start talking to each other, the real stuff will come to the surface. The things you've been wanting to talk about but didn't have a chance to because you've been tired or because you've been fighting a lot and you feel defeated. It happens. Start communicating about what's been on your mind, the things you'd like to see differently or the emotions that have been building up. The fog will clear and you will see what you've been wanting to talk about or what you've been hiding subconsciously. Once you've started talking together, you'll feel a lot better and you two will probably grow closer again. Just take the first step, despite how scary it might seem.

Invest in each other

You're investing in your relationship each time you organize a date night. But you can invest in your relationship daily, in smaller ways. For example, give your partner a compliment every now and then. Try to remember the things you loved about your partner when you first met. Or remember how things were between you two before you had a baby.

Yes, it sounds simple, but it really works. Be positive toward your partner, and don't forget that postpartum is not a walk in the park for them, either. Yes, you're the star of the show because you gave birth to the baby and you've done an incredible job throughout the entire pregnancy and birth. However, your partner was there too, most likely worrying, and deserves your loving attention and compliments now and again.

Give each other a hug, a pat on the back, or a spontaneous kiss on a regular basis. Tiny gestures like remembering to stock up on your partner's favourite snack can make a big difference and help reassure them that they're still important to you, that it's not just about the baby. Start looking for things that connect you. The more common ground you find, the better. It can be small things, but let them be there. It will make you bond more as a couple and you two will remember who you were before you became parents. Of course, your partner has to return the favour. If you have a partner who isn't always the thoughtful type, learn to ask for what you need directly. Some dads find they lose their wife when she becomes a mother. She only has eyes for the baby now, which can make some fathers feel neglected or flat-out ignored. These feelings are valid and should be addressed. So, dad, if you're reading this, start opening up about your thoughts and feelings, even if you're not used to doing so and the thought of it makes you feel very awkward. Communication is everything. It's normal that you need to find a new balance once the baby is here.

When your partner feels like you haven't been paying a lot of attention to him or her, please listen. You both want the same thing: to be loved and to be heard. By taking each other's feelings seriously, you're already showing how much you care. Put some effort into letting your partner know that he or she still matters to you. That despite the fact that you're a mother now, the old version of you is still in there and that you still care for your partner deeply. A relationship is hard work sometimes. There are couples who pretend that this is not the case, I wouldn't take them too seriously. Rremember that just because the relationship can be hard work doesn't mean that there's anything wrong with it. Ups and downs are completely normal.

The hard work in your relationship is also about being kind to each other. Make both of you responsible for your relationship. One of my friends told me her partner pointed out that she was checking up on him all the time. She was checking if he did the dishes right, folded the laundry the right way, and if he had bought the right type of bread. The first thing she did upon coming home from work was to tour the house to see if he had done everything according to her routine. Understandably, it drove him crazy and put a big strain on their relationship. They hashed it out in the end. This couple worked hard to get through their difficulties by talking, going to therapy together, and communicating in a positive way. Of course, sometimes one of the two pulls the cart a little harder than the other one. That, too, has to balance itself out. What I am trying to say is, make time for each other, invest in each other, and treat each other with respect and love.

Insecurity

My American girlfriend told me about her postpartum depression. She was convinced that her husband was cheating on her with a younger, smarter version of herself. Every day she asked him if he still loved her. It can be really hard to be on the receiving end of this, to feel that your other half questions your love so regularly. I urged my friend to talk to her husband about her worries, about feeling unattractive with a postpartum belly and the healing wound in her vagina. Eventually she told her husband that she couldn't imagine him still finding her pretty or sexy. Her husband responded in a deeply reassuring way. He hugged her and said, "Listen, you're my wife, the mother of our child. I wouldn't trade you for anyone else." Talking to her husband and opening up about her insecurities really helped her get over the self-doubt that she'd been bottling up for months. Keeping any worry inside makes it a lot worse. So many women feel insecure after giving birth, about their body, motherhood, etc. If you build it all up inside, you'll most likely slip into a negative spiral. My friend saw her negative feelings gradually disappear after she started to communicate her fears and jealous thoughts to her husband. It just needs time, dear moms, but you, too, will get through this!

Back in the day, I told my husband that I wanted to feel like the old Tilda again, both inside and out. That I'd imagined life as a mother so differently and that I hoped he still saw me as *his* Tilda, not just as a mommy with leaking tits. I asked him if he still found me attractive and if he was happy with me, despite everything that was going on. He replied, "Yes, of course, darling, I love you so much." He had to get used to the new me as well. During sex my boobs leaked milk. I mean, that was a bit of a shocker for him. Tim laughingly told me he didn't just love me for my perky breasts. He loved me for who I truly was, the way I made him laugh until he cried, how I made him feel, our shared history. None of that had disappeared just because my breasts weren't looking their finest.

What do you do when you're a single mom and you don't have a significant other to reassure you? This is very hard, because all new moms need validation at some point. I would advise you to look for a single parent support group. Or try to connect with friends or acquaintances who also have kids. You might find a welcoming online community of parents who are single, just like you. Try to find reassurance and comfort in friends who get you. Being a single mother can be incredibly hard, and I applaud you for doing this alone. You're a superhero.

What do you do if your partner isn't supportive, or you feel that they're no longer attracted to you? A client found herself in a marriage without affection. Her husband didn't show her any love. He didn't give her a single hug or kiss, let alone a compliment. She was devastated. Their sex life was nonexistent, and her self-esteem had left the building as well. I advised her to be honest with her partner, to tell him that the relationship wasn't working for her. She was very nervous and had to build up to it. But they sat down one night and talked for hours. She cried a lot during that conversation and her partner finally got it. He was actually very apologetic once he could see things from her point of view. He was just overwhelmed by the responsibilities of new fatherhood and was having a very hard time himself, which she wouldn't have known if they hadn't had that conversation. In the end, they made things work.

CHAPTER 13

Let's Talk about Sex

Sex is like sleeping
I'm not doing
Enough of
Either of them

Those first weeks after giving birth are all about healing. Your body and mind are processing the experience. This requires time and patience. Most women need some time adapting to a new body and that's normal. Just do what feels right for you. Better yet, please don't do anything you don't feel comfortable with, and trust your intuition when it comes to sex.

Having sex might be the last thing on your mind when you're so busy taking care of your newborn. Or maybe you're really keen but your partner isn't ready. Please know there is no right or wrong. As a couple you need to recalibrate. And then there's the fact that sex is obviously quite a big deal when you're recovering from having giving birth because it involves your state of mind *and* your vagina, both which have taken quite a battering.

My first time

I wasn't too keen on having sex for the first time after having Liv. I was in the deepest and darkest pit I'd ever been in. Sex was the last thing on my mind. At the same time, I was well aware of the fact that Tim wanted to, and I didn't want to disappoint him. I remember it all very clearly. I had my six-week check-up with my ob-gyn and she made me look at my foof. She told me that I might as well look now and promised me that it wasn't that bad. I honestly didn't want to look. Not because I'm prudish or shy, but because I simply didn't want to be reminded of the traumatic birth experience. It was traumatic because my epidural was shut down as soon as I needed to push and I was in intense pain in a matter of minutes. Then, I had to push for two hours and she wouldn't come out. To top it all off, they stitched me back up without any anesthetics. It was tough. That scar down there brought it all back. It still makes me emotional, remembering this all. But she was insistent, and I didn't dare argue with a medical professional. So I just lay there with that mirror clamped between my hands and I remember feeling awful, that I'd been brutalized.

After that check-up, I went home, adamant that I was going to have sex with my husband. The ob-gyn had given me the all clear. I was semi-excited to be able to reconnect on that level with my husband, but I was also very nervous. I certainly didn't feel a wave of desire, but I did feel the need to reconnect with him. Despite the depression, the sleep deprivation, I wanted our relationship to go back to how it once was. Just be Tim and Tilda again. Needless to say, Tim was *very* excited. When we put Livia to bed, we lit some candles, played romantic music, and dimmed the lights. I felt so insecure about my body that I would have preferred we turn off all the lights. Sex in the dark seemed a pretty good idea. So we started and I felt nervous. He was also a little tense but mostly thrilled. After a while I started to notice a sharp, cutting pain in my pelvic area. I say pelvic area, because I couldn't tell exactly where the pain was coming from. (I now know it was from my episiotomy scar.) I tried to ignore the pain but it intensified, so we paused. I asked him if he'd forgotten to cut his fingernails. He hadn't, so we tried again and it still hurt. We stopped and I felt like an utter failure. I cried and cried and felt like I was the biggest disappointment ever. Why couldn't I make this work? My husband was very sweet but a bit clumsy with what he said. He meant well but it wasn't that helpful. In the end I got out of bed and went into the bathroom. I took a long shower and texted my best friend about how much a disappointment the whole thing had been. She texted me back. Two words: lube gel. Very practical advice!

I talked to my mom friend and she advised me to wait another six weeks before trying again, which I thought sounded sensible. I spoke to Tim and six weeks later, I stocked up on lube gel and we were good to go. Finally, we could have sex without pain. I was so relieved and actually enjoyed sex again. We kept using the lube gel for a couple of months. After I quit breastfeeding, my body went back to normal and the mucous membranes did what they're supposed to do. I'd advise everyone to get lube gel and use it when you're dry down there. When I gave birth to Emmi it was completely different. I didn't put any pressure on myself, and because of that I avoided the whole crying and feeling like a failure situation. This time, I felt ready for sex before the six-week check-up, although I still waited to be sure. I think it was easier the second time because of the non-traumatic labour. Also, I didn't have PPD.

It's important to take time to recover after the birth of your baby, which is why you'll probably be advised to not have inter-course within six weeks after the birth. After six weeks, the cervix is usually properly closed and any stitches have dissolved, so the risk of infection is reduced. Sex after the birth is certainly not advisable while you're still bleeding. On average, the flow stops three to six weeks after giving birth. In those weeks you still have a chance of getting infections, so it's definitely not wise to have sex. Then after six weeks you can slowly start trying to have sex again, but don't rush it.

Maybe you're feeling like, *Oh, yeah! Finally, I can have sex again!* Or maybe it's the last thing you want to think about. Both reactions and everything in between is completely fine and normal. From my experience, most moms aren't even thinking about having sex so soon after delivery, but their partners often are, which can put a lot of pressure on the new mother. "Should I be having sex with my partner, even though I'm not ready?" a client once asked me. My answer was, *'No!'*

While it's understandable that you want to score some (major) points with your partner, you don't want to force yourself into doing anything that doesn't feel comfortable. Your body needs a proper six weeks to heal. Some mothers have stitches; other mothers have a stage 4 rupture of the perineum. The last thing you want to do is force a penis in there. I can't stress this enough: You don't have to have sex if you feel you're not ready. Feeling a little nervous is natural. But when you feel really anxious, wait another couple of weeks. And just because your ob-gyn says you can have sex, you obviously still don't have to. Of course, you can try and it might go very well. There's also a possibility that it doesn't feel right yet, in which case just stop.

Dr Eveline Stallaart, a sexologist based in the Netherlands, says, 'Don't have sex before the six-week check-up. Some mothers present it as something cool, that they "couldn't wait" to have sex again. Please know that you risk a serious infection doing that.'

Set the bar low

There are all sorts of reasons that sex after birth is a bit more complicated than the enjoyable romp it used to be. For some women, they're just as afraid about having sex again as they'd be having their wisdom teeth removed. For some other women it's like they jump back in the saddle like nothing ever happened. Either way, sex *will* be different. As an ob-gyn friend once told me, 'When you have sex again after having children, it could feel like you're throwing a banana down the hallway.'

Right.

I'm just gonna leave that there…

According to Dr Eveline Stallaart, the expectations are often too high. 'For a long time, everything was dominated by the idea that something had to get out of your vagina, and now suddenly something has to go in. You had to wait six weeks to have sex again. In the meantime, your attention mostly goes to your new child and your different life. Hormones make it harder to get sexually aroused, and there's a good chance that you'll have trouble getting wet. As the partner, you've been patient for a long time and there's often a need to be intimate together again, but how do you start? It's often expected that it will be like before immediately, but with all these changes, how could that be the case?'

Some moms feel rather discouraged after trying to have sex for the first time after childbirth. This is often because they set the bar far too high for themselves. I think that the first time should be some sort of a test drive to see how your foof is feeling and if she likes something going in there again. If she doesn't, just stop and try again in another couple of weeks. It's okay, really! A number of women don't enjoy sex postpartum right away. Is that a bad thing? No. Trust me, you'll enjoy it again. You just need to get used to and trust your body again after all it's been through. For some women that takes only six weeks postpartum, for others (like me) it took three to four months, and for yet another group of moms it might take nine months. Take your time and don't force yourself to do anything you don't want. It might take some trying and getting used to again, but that's understandable. I mean, you pushed a watermelon through your nose. Can it get any more brutal?

It's important to realize that the first time you have sex again after childbirth is not representative of what your sex life is going to be like forever. Your foof has been stretched (hello baby) and bruised or maybe even cut open. That is traumatic to the entire pelvic area. Your vagina needs time to heal and you need to recover mentally.

For me, the road back to having sex after my first baby was complicated. I didn't trust my body. The birth was intense. I had a huge hematoma pressing on my episiotomy scar and I couldn't sit, walk, or stand up straight without a lot of pain. Just thinking about sex made me want to gag, honestly. After the six-week check-up, my scar had healed nicely and I was given the all-clear to start working out again and having sex. I think I subconsciously felt pressure. I'd been cleared for sex, but should I? I definitely wanted to try again, but now, right away? In retrospect, I probably should have waited. Our second attempt was better: no pain and a big relief that it worked out. Both of us were happy we tried. Was it great sex? No. But that came along. We just kept going and by the time Liv was nine months old, it felt like the old days again. My scar would sometimes be sensitive and it sometimes still is. But it wasn't painful anymore. Enjoying sex again is so important for your relationship.

Partners

It may be that your partner is ready for sex earlier than you are. That happens a lot and it's important to not feel pressured into anything. Remember that there's more to sex than just penetration. Try other fun things first. And there's also more to intimacy than sexual activity. If you're not ready for any kind of sexual contact, maybe think about nonsexual physical ways you can reach out to your partner. Long hugs can feel amazing, for example, and can also feel reassuring. As long as you keep talking to each other, you'll often work it out together. Communication is key in every relationship.

Some people might find talking about sex uncomfortable. They just do it (or don't) but they don't necessarily want to talk about it. As understandable as that might be, communication about a sensitive matter such as sex is important for a healthy relationship. When you're open and honest about what you're going through, there will likely be fewer misunderstandings between the two of you. If you tell your partner honestly about how scared you are to have sex again and that it has nothing to do with him or her, they won't feel offended or insecure. They could be disappointed, but that's perfectly okay; they're allowed to have those feelings. Not being ready for sex right now doesn't mean that you won't be ready ever. It's a temporary situation. Please share this with your partner, too. Tell them how you feel and ask them to trust you and to have patience and that you will tell them when you're ready. Every woman, every mother needs her own time to get into the groove again. If you notice that after nine to twelve months you still have difficulties or pain during sex, please visit your doctor and ask for help. You deserve all the help you can get.

Another possibility is that it's your partner who doesn't feel the need for sex yet. Some partners may be feeling rejected, a little bit like they're the third wheel in the relationship. Some might suffer from images they saw during the birth. They've experienced a very different function of the vagina, and switching back to seeing the sexual side of the vagina again can sometimes be difficult. It's possible that some partners no longer see their wives as sexual. In my experience, this definitely subsides, and they'll get over it soon enough! My husband was there all the way during the delivery of both our kids. He needed some adjustment period after both deliveries, that's for sure. He's also brutally honest, and trust me, that's not always what I needed from him. But we got back to normal and he started to see me and treat me as a sexual human being again. With most partners the (traumatic) images of the birth subside after a few weeks. Ultimately, both you and your partner should be able to see your vagina again as 'sexual' so you can start enjoying sex again. If your partner still has trouble digesting what he or she saw during the birth, please ask for help. Like I said before, if things aren't back to the way they used to be nine to twelve months postpartum, please see your doctor and start looking for a therapist.

Practical tips: If you're squeamish, look away now!

Dryness is a problem postpartum. I just want to get this out there. For some reason that I can't possibly fathom, women don't seem to talk about this much. A friend of mine told me about when she tried having sex again for the first time after giving birth. She put in all the work, shaving her legs for the first time in a month. She also shaved her armpits and foof, because you know, once you get going, you might as well go all the way. She bought a new negligee—not lingerie, because she got too depressed by the lighting in the fitting room. After taking her baby to her parents' house, she drove home, listening to some '90s rap and R&B to get in the mood. She came home all cheerful and confident. Her husband was on his way from work and she lit the candles, even the scented ones. All the lights were on dim mode and she did her hair and put on some mascara. You could say she was *ready*.

When her husband came home, she practically jumped on him. He was surprised but very into it. They went to the bedroom, started to make out, and he was super excited. So they tried to have sex. But she was dry. So dry, his penis couldn't enter at all. This was a massive shock to my friend, because she was obviously aroused, as was he, but that didn't equal successful intercourse. They didn't have any lubricant on hand, so they tried and tried but it wouldn't work out. My friend called me in tears half an hour later. I felt so sad for her. Her husband tried to comfort her, telling her that it was okay, but she could feel his disappointment as well. I told her that it was all very normal but that nobody talks about it. The dryness is a result of hormonal changes, not something you can do or change. I told her that it wasn't her fault and that it would be better next time. I advised her to buy some good lube gel and go for it again in a couple of days. She did, and it was a success. She was feeling so relieved after this and she and her partner thanked me later.

Thanks to those hormonal changes, pretty much every woman experiences some level of dryness down there postpartum. The levels of oestrogen and progesterone drop significantly after the birth. The female body decreases the oestrogen level further while a mother is nursing because oestrogen can hinder milk production. Oestrogen is very important for sexual arousal. If you have reduced levels of it you can experience symptoms similar to women who go through menopause, including hot flashes, night sweats, and vaginal dryness. I had all those symptoms after giving birth. It was unreal. I absolutely hated it. You can take an oestrogen supplement to help you with this, although there may be some associated health risks. Please discuss it with your doctor.

The first thing you want to do is buy a good lubricant gel. One that feels nice, maybe a scented one. I wouldn't go for the complicated versions that give you a tingling foof. I mean, there's enough going on as it is. Normal lubricant will suffice. Warm the gel between your hands so your foof doesn't get scared of the coldness coming her way. We want her enthusiastic, not timid. Once you've warmed up the gel, place it in and around your vagina. Also, put some gel on his penis, so you're both nice and smooth to begin with. Remember, if it doesn't feel right, you can always quit. Bear in mind that the first time you have sex after delivery, the entire penis might not fit in completely. This might seem counterintuitive, because a baby fit through there, right? However, your vagina had some serious trauma to digest and might be less elastic then normal. Lower oestrogen levels can cause urogenital atrophy, including epithelial thinning but also decreased elasticity and diminished vaginal blood flow. No wonder having sex for the first time can be a challenge. Just guide the penis in with your hand and if it hurts, just say, 'Stop.'

As I've said, it's always a good idea to talk about it with your partner first. I know, it might feel awkward and totally not sexy, but your partner needs to know what they can expect, too. Remember, you will have sex again and you will enjoy it again. Every woman is different and every vagina is different. So be gentle with yourself.

Everything is different

Even an orgasm may feel different after giving birth. This is because your womb is still very sensitive. Orgasms can therefore be more intense; sometimes better, sometimes worse. Having an orgasm can even hurt a little. Don't worry, this usually passes and at some point, you'll no longer experience any pain. It's impossible to say when exactly that will happen, but if you have severe pain or the pain hasn't gone away after nine to twelve months, please go to the doctor.

Dr Eveline Stallaart says, 'Pain always means stop right away! It's a sign from your body that you're not quite there yet, with your head. Don't try to act tough and don't fight through the pain, but listen to your body. You might want to try and extend the foreplay or wait a while before penetration. If the pain continues to occur, go to your doctor.'

If you've had a C-section, things can also feel different, too. Your womb has been cut open and stitched back together. So when you have an orgasm, you can feel that particular area. This is nothing to worry about and it will pass or at least get less noticeable.

Your Kegel muscles can get a little lazy after you've given birth, so orgasms may be harder to achieve those first weeks or months. Trust your body and know that this also will get better. You just need to do your Kegel exercises again. It helps tremendously. I did Kegels before I was pregnant, too. I read about it and felt I wanted to prepare myself for a pregnancy in the future. I still do the exercises now. They really strengthen the pelvic floor and can be helpful to avoid or minimize incontinence. I recommend doing them as often as you can. I'm doing mine as I write ;).

If you've had to squeeze a mini person through your vagina, you may have had a tear or episiotomy. At first, the area down under no longer resembles what it was. It may look black and blue or like a butcher has been at work. Please don't panic! Your vagina is well supplied with blood and recovers with time. Fair enough, there's a chance that it will never be *quite* the same as before. You may notice the changes and maybe your partner will, too. Most women don't ask their spouses, the subject being a taboo thing. I think most women learn to accept their new body eventually, but for some it's more challenging than others. When you do decide to take that mirror and take a peek down under, don't worry if your vagina not only looks different but also has a slightly different colour than before. Due to the hormonal changes in your body, your vagina usually gets a little darker but will return to your original colour when your hormones stabilize. Sometimes not. Again, it's all normal!

Flooding

In the Netherlands, home births are very common, and every pregnant woman receives a maternity package from her health insurance in case she delivers her baby at home. Any woman who opens her maternity package before giving birth has a lovely surprise: *enormous* sanitary pads. They're most certainly not sexy, but they're useful. After giving birth you're likely to suffer from a light to severe 'maternity flood'. This can last for about six weeks. And as if this long period isn't enough, the 'flood' can smell a bit strange, sometimes Tes even fishy. If it smells very unpleasant, go to the doctor to rule out an infection. I remember leaking a bit during sex. I wasn't sure what was happening, but I tried to stay calm and carried on having sex. Sometimes Kegels will help with this issue.

Even after the smoothest delivery, you might well experience a certain amount of pain when sitting, when you're urinating or wiping. This too will pass. Tip: If you don't have an AquaClean toilet at home, use a jug of water; it works well as a temporary alternative to toilet paper or in case of pain while urinating because it thins the urine and makes it feel less prickly.

Birth control

Almost everyone knows of someone who got pregnant again within a few weeks or months of giving birth. The fact is that you can be fertile again really quickly after childbirth, even if you're breastfeeding and don't have your period. There are so many myths out there about fertility after childbirth, but I strongly recommend relying on contraception if you don't want to get pregnant again right away. Talk to your doctor about your options and which one might suit you best.

CHAPTER 14

Travelling: Babies Are Super Portable

Travelling is about
Finding things
You never knew
You were looking for

Mothers who don't feel well after childbirth tend to stay at home. It's just easier to be away from all stimuli and confrontations with the outside world. If you're one of these women, the thought of travelling may fill you with horror. If you can barely cope at home, a holiday can feel downright terrifying. *What if he cries for the entire flight? What if he won't sleep once we're there?* The idea of letting go of the routine and structure you've created at home can feel scary to a lot of new parents. In this chapter you'll read why it doesn't have to be this way and how to make travel not only easier but also fun.

I found going on a trip even though I was feeling very low to be really healing. I highly recommend it. You get away from your day-to-day routines that might be making you feel trapped. You'll have a change of scene and you'll meet new people. It can also work wonders for your relationship and your sense of self. You have more time for self-care (meditation, for example) because you aren't swamped by your normal daily activities. Travelling can also put things in perspective. Maybe things aren't as bad as you've been picturing them in your head. And I always get the most creative ideas while on vacation. It is like my mind opens up and I have space for brand-new ideas. When you realize you *can* cope with your new baby no matter where you are, it will do a lot for your self-esteem. And last but not least, when you travel, you realize your life isn't over just because you've had a baby. This can be very inspiring. Add some good weather, good food, and a break from the day-to-day routine, and you have all the ingredients for feeling a bit better.

My story

When Livia was seven months old, we decided it was time to go on a vacation. To South Africa. It sounds a bit crazy, doesn't it? Take one very depressed woman, one brand-new baby, and add an exhausted partner, and put them together on a 10-hour flight. A recipe for disaster, surely?

For as long as my husband and I have been together, we've enjoyed going on adventurous holidays. We planned to continue to do so even after we had children. Of course, we hadn't anticipated PPD. But despite the depression, it turned out that I needed a vacation more than anything else at that point. My life for the previous seven months had been dominated by depression and anxiety, but when we went on holiday, the old me slowly resurfaced. Travelling through South Africa felt like coming home. We had such a wonderful time reconnecting with the country. We went back to where we got married and reconnected with all the lovely people there. It was so heart-warming. I felt like my old self again. Bringing back all these memories from our wedding was amazing and being there with our baby who we proudly showed to everyone was fantastic. The old Tilda peeked over the fence. Just a tiny bit. I felt so grateful. I had felt the old me was lost forever.

Before we went on the trip, I felt incredibly stressed. I lay in bed at night, imagining how disastrous that long flight could be. Would it go well? Would Liv's ears be painful during take-off and landing? Would she cry for the entire flight? You name it, I worried about it. I talked to Tim about it (a lot) and he said, 'We've travelled so much together in the past, under way more stressful circumstances. I don't see why we can't pull this off.' This made sense to me and I felt slightly reassured. I also talked to my therapist about it. She thought it was a great idea and encouraged us to go.

None of my doom scenarios happened during the flight. In fact, she cried only once during that 10-hour flight to Cape Town. Once! She mostly slept or played nicely in her basket, which the flight attendants had attached to the wall in front of us. We were sitting in the bulkhead seats, which I can highly recommend.

Of course, I can't guarantee that you'll have the same experience. One thing we know about babies is that they're going to do their own thing. The best-laid plans can go awry. The key is to be able to laugh at 'disaster' journeys. Since that first easy trip, I've had flights with challenging moments with both our girls. Once, Emmi decided that sleep was so very 2016 and refused to so much as shut an eye. Liv was wide awake, too, but could at least be entertained with a Disney movie. A few hours into that flight, both Tim and I were exhausted. It was 2 a.m. and I could barely keep my eyes open. Tim held Emmi and I had Liv on my lap. I felt my head drop every two minutes. At some point Tim took them both so I could have a nap. An hour later we reversed. Needless to say, we were complete zombies when we left the plane. I think we could have auditioned for the TV show 'The Walking Dead' and they would have loved to have us. Very convincing characters. After stressful flights, where one of the girls cried or didn't seem to listen to anything we said, I have to shake off the thoughts in my head that everyone must think I'm a bad mother. In all likelihood, you'll never see these passengers again, and once you've arrived at your destination, chances are that you'll forget about the journey in no time.

If you've had a difficult trip, for whatever reason, accept that it didn't work out as you had hoped, and let it go. Worrying in advance isn't going to change the outcome. It's a waste of time and energy because ultimately there's only so much you can control. Your baby has a mind of her own. Try to accept that you can't control any of it and then let the negative thoughts and emotions go, just as I described in the chapter about mindfulness. Travelling with a baby is a really great opportunity to put your mindfulness skills into practice!

The benefits of going on holiday

It may well be the last thing you want to think about, but I'm going to keep banging on about it: Going on holiday can really help you through your PPD or general low mood. It forces you to step out of your comfort zone (often your own house) and go out into the wide world with your baby. It can be super fun to see how she reacts to the big new world out there, and you, too, will have new and positive experiences that are likely to improve your mood, at least temporarily.

I remember introducing Livia to the ocean that first holiday. We thought she'd love it and be desperate to splash about. As soon as we walked into the sea with Liv in Tim's arms, she started to whine a little. We didn't know this was fear; we thought she was getting excited. Little did we know. Tim lowered her to ocean level and tried to dip her little feet in the water. She was screaming now. Literally crying at the top of her lungs. We were like, 'Okay, so this wasn't a great idea.' I did enjoy the moment, though. It was our first family vacay and I was so happy being there. We stuck to a swimming pool after that, which Liv absolutely loved. She wasn't afraid of the water, but the sound and intensity of the waves probably scared her (and sometimes still does). We swam together and she laughed the entire time. I felt so proud. We did it. We flew to the other side of the world and were enjoying ourselves so much with our baby girl. Not only that, but it also really boosted my self-confidence as a parent. That's how it went down for us. When the long flight was over, we'd say positive things to each other such as 'We did a great job together!'

Travelling together as a couple (or alone with your baby) has other perks. It can do wonders for your relationship with whomever you're travelling with, be it a partner or friend. You can reconnect on a deeper level with each other. This is hard in a society that demands so much from us. While you normally might only have snatched moments together in the daily grind, during your holiday you have hours per day where you can talk, laugh, and interact. It doesn't get better than that. Going on holiday with a baby is also about finding your identity again, because you see that your life doesn't stop just because you've become a mother.

You also broaden your horizons when it comes to culture, food, and a new language. Learning new things and using your brain in a different way is great for creativity, helping us find new ways of looking at things or problem solving. All of this is great when you're not on cloud nine; you might get a new idea for how to solve a problem, or you might find a new interest you can pick up once you're back home.

I remember one specific moment when we were on vacation with our daughter for the first time. I was half asleep and when I properly woke up, I sat up and said, 'It's almost scary to admit it, but I'm actually starting to feel happy again.' It was a huge revelation to me and a big turning point in my life. I hadn't felt well, let alone happy, for months and months. Deciding to go on vacation despite my postpartum depression felt like a big risk.

Our friends and family had been hesitant about our plans. But we both really wanted to go, so we ignored all the well-meaning comments and off we flew to Cape Town. It felt like a huge mountain to climb, even though a holiday is something that's supposed to be fun! In the lead up to the holiday, I lost count of how many times I doubted whether we should do it or not. I kept thinking, *I can't do this!*

If you're feeling the same, I have good news for you. Yes, you can! I promise, you can. Below, you'll find some tips that can help make things a little easier.

What if it doesn't feel possible?

Maybe you really doubt you can pull off a holiday. Maybe it doesn't feel like a realistic goal at all. That's totally fine. You don't have to do anything you don't want to do. But a change of scenery might do you some good. So, if you're hesitant, let me help you out. One of my clients asked me for tips, because she thought the stress of planning and packing would make her feel worse.

First of all, acknowledge that it's perfectly normal to feel this way. Every new parent will feel nervous about flying or travelling with their child for the first time. Start by making a list of what to pack. Do it with plenty of time to spare, so when you suddenly remember something, you can just add it to the list. It's most convenient to make the packing list digital, so you can re-use it for every trip. I also made individual lists for Livia and Emmi, and I amend them each year, because they grow up so fast. Do some fun research. There are online routes, maps, and travel plans everywhere you look.

Another client wondered if she should even go on holiday, because she didn't have a partner.

Of course you can go! I totally get why you could be hesitant, but you have options. You could go with friend(s), your sister, or your mother. You should choose someone you feel comfortable with and who loves to be with you and your baby. And then if you want to explore the town in the evening, or go to a local yoga class, your travelling companion can babysit. If you don't feel comfortable with this, you could also go on holiday alone. Start small, do something fun together, and when that goes well, you can do a weekend away, then a full holiday. Or maybe you're feeling brave already and want to fly across the Atlantic with your baby. That's all good!

My friend who is on a tight budget asked me how she should handle a holiday.

You can start small and do day trips, city breaks, etc. Maybe you know a friend in another city/state/country you could ask if you can stay overnight (or longer) with them. There's also the option of a house swap. That way you can save up for the fun stuff and won't break the bank on the accommodation.

Some of my clients told me they didn't want to go outside their comfort zone too much. They'd just had a baby and felt like a trip was just too much. I always advise women to start with baby steps. You don't have to travel half the world. Just do what feels right for you.

Taking your depressed mind on holiday

If you're on holiday and you find yourself suddenly hit by depressive thoughts or anxiety attacks, please know that this doesn't mean your whole trip is ruined. You can have these thoughts and still be mostly okay; you can have some difficult moments and it still will have been a really worthwhile trip. Look over the section on mindfulness in chapter 5. Please do the metaphor exercise again and again, visualizing any negative thoughts or emotions drifting away. Accept that the situation is what it is. You can try to flee from it or fight it, but doing that will cost you so much more energy than if you just accept it. Every mother is different, and every day is different. Take each day as it comes and accept your response to the situations life will throw at you.

When you notice something pleasing, be it a beautiful view or the sound of your baby chuckling, take a good few seconds to appreciate it, to notice everything you can about that moment. Take it all in. These moments help interrupt the negative cycle of your postpartum depression. Of course, the stifling grey cloud will not disappear right away, but at times you're likely to feel much better than if you had been stuck at home all day.

Pay attention to what went well. It's so easy to focus on the negatives, but celebrating the good things improves your mood greatly. During your vacation you'll do all sorts of fun things, discover beautiful places, and meet new people. Although these can help distract you, they're unlikely to 'cure' your depression. My fears most certainly didn't vanish because we switched continents. But despite those fears, I was able to enjoy many moments we had as a new family of three. The holiday definitely improved my mental state. When we got home, I was a bit afraid that I would slip back into depressive mode. I asked myself on the plane, *What if I can't hold on to these positive feelings? What if I spiral back into depression?* But once we got home, I noticed that I continued feeling mostly more positive. I had moments of feeling low again, but I could remember some of the fun memories from our travels and found more of a sense that the depression wouldn't last forever. Everything changes and I knew that this depression wasn't going to last until the end of time. My therapist noticed the changes, too. She saw a different Tilda.

Tips and tricks: what to pack

Blackout fabric

My must-have item for travel with children is a piece of blackout material. It sounds a bit dramatic, but nothing is more annoying than being awake at 5 a.m. after your child has finally fallen asleep but not being able to sleep yourself because the hotel curtains are transparent. Also carry tape and safety pins in that same bag, so you have everything you need to immediately darken the windows on arrival. And you can all go to sleep soundly after a long journey.

A stroller with a reclining seat

This is really useful because it means you have a portable cot and won't have to rush back to your accommodation whenever it's nap time. I'd put a muslin over the stroller to stimulate 'nap time', and meanwhile Tim and I could have lunch.

It's important to know that only small and collapsible strollers are allowed to travel to the door of the airplane. Bigger strollers have to be checked in. I prefer to travel with a smaller stroller so I don't have to carry babies through the airport! With a small stroller, you can walk everywhere and put your hand luggage in it or hang your bags on it. Plus, your baby can sleep in it comfortably. Double win.

Hand luggage: clean sets of clothing and a large muslin

No matter how old your child is, a few large muslins are incredibly useful. You can wrap your child in it, you can use it as a burp cloth, make a cover out of it, and even wrap yourself in it when breastfeeding, if that's what you prefer. An extra set of clothes are handy, too, because for some reason babies can suddenly have an exploding diaper at high altitude. Roll up a t-shirt for yourself and put it in the diaper bag. You don't want to know how often I was spat up on or pooped on during a flight… It feels great to freshen up afterward and put on a clean t-shirt!

Bring a replica of baby's favourite soft toy

It's highly likely that your child's favourite animal must go everywhere with her. It's very sweet, but it can make some parents anxious of the drama if the animal gets lost. My advice is to buy a replica of her favourite toy or blanket and put it in your own hand luggage, so you always have one to hand. No deafening tears and inconsolable baby if Doodoo is left in Terminal 3.

Tips and tricks: the journey

Make a few phone calls in advance

There are some unavoidable unknowns when you go on holiday, and I think the most important thing you can do is to realize that you can't control everything. Having said that, I'd recommend a phone call to the airline and an email to the hotel/accommodation before you go.

Whether you've decided to go camping at a family-friendly site or you're going to a hotel in Thailand, e-mail them in advance to check whether they have a baby bed/cot and ask them to set it up in the room before you arrive. This avoids you having to wait for the baby cot to be found when you've just arrived, tired and wanting to settle down.

Try and request bulkhead seats for your flights. These are the seats immediately behind the walls on an airplane that separate the sections. These are the seats that everyone wants but almost never gets. The ones with extra legroom. Don't wait until you get to the airport to request these seats, but call the airline a few months in advance, or set a timer for the earliest possible opportunity you can check in online. I think bulkhead seats are a life saver. Thanks to the extra legroom, your child has a place to sit and play, and in the meantime you can relax, because your baby isn't continuously on your lap.

If there aren't any bulkhead seats available, I'd still recommend letting the airline know that you're travelling with a baby, and asking whether the seat(s) next to you can be left free if the flight isn't full. Airlines tend to be pretty accommodating because they don't want a crying baby on a long-haul flight any more than you do. Ask again when you get to the airport and go to the airport extra early to avoid stress and rushing.

You will probably worry about everything that could possibly go wrong during the trip or flight. Using your mindfulness skills, practice watching letting those thoughts float away. Notice if you're afraid of what fellow travellers might think about you. Remember that many of these people have been or one day will be in your situation. Most people understand that you don't want your baby to cry during a flight. And also bear in mind you'll probably never see these people again and you don't have to feel guilty or ashamed. After the flight you say goodbye and that's it.

Find a quiet corner at the airport

Once I'm checked in, I like to find a corner of the airport that's a bit quieter, somewhere perfect for breastfeeding or quietening your baby down. Walk around calmly, and before you know it, you'll spot a good place. Sometimes, you can find sockets there so you can recharge your phone or tablet. A large scarf at the bottom of the stroller can offer a solution as a shield against stimuli. If your stroller has a reclining seat, your child can take a nice nap in it. If it's not nap time, then maybe you and she can go to a window and watch airplanes together. That's a fun activity, especially when they get older. Watching the planes taking off and landing together is very exciting! Many airports have play areas for children, which are super useful for when your little one isn't napping and wants to play. I love those playgrounds inside airports. Your child can get rid of her extra energy and you can sit and relax a bit.

Shift work

What I really like to do while travelling with Tim and the kids, be it by car or plane, is to divide the trip into shifts. For example, your partner/travel companion can drive for four hours and then you switch over. On the plane, your partner does all the snacks, bottles, diapers, and naps for the first half, and you do the entire second half of the flight. That way you can take turns sleeping or just being able to switch off. This is especially nice during night flights, so you can both get some sleep.

Relax the rules

The tablet or phone is your best friend during a long journey. You can load up a tablet with fun videos and your baby's favourite games. I don't usually allow a lot of screen time on regular days, but during a long trip, the rules go out of the window. It simply makes no sense to have rigid rules during a long and tiring journey with an overtired toddler. Be nice to yourself! After the flight, you can pick up your regular rules about screen or TV time again and your kids will be back in their old routine.

You don't have to take a pile of toys on board. Your baby is likely to find everything on the plane fascinating, because it's all new. She'll be amazed by the table in front of you that can open and close, and by the window from which she can stare endlessly. On one particularly relaxing flight, Liv played for hours with the earplugs we got from the flight attendants. She lay on the floor between our feet and played with them, really content.

Tips and tricks: once you're there

The first night will be the hardest, but don't panic

Just like us, your baby will have to get used to her new environment, her new bed. She may also be overwhelmed by the stimuli during a long journey, which might mean she won't go to sleep right away. Try not to panic. It doesn't mean that every night of your trip will be like this. From my experience, things go back to normal after the first two nights. If not, and your baby isn't sleeping during the night, try to split the night into shifts, as I suggested you do on flights. You'll all be sleeping in the same room, so take ear plugs with you. There's no need for you both to be awake all night. It might help to bring your baby's favourite blanket, cuddle bear, etc., anything to make her feel at home far away from home.

Start an evening ritual

I recommend starting an evening ritual as soon as possible and then continuing that ritual as best you can while you're on holiday. It could be anything you and your baby like: the same song, the same bedtime story after the bath. The options are endless, so choose something that suits you and your child. This way she will start to recognize the bedtime routine and realize when it's time for bed. She's likely to fall asleep faster, because she understands what needs to be done: sleeping. We did this right after our daughter was born, but you can start at any time.

I even recreated the routine on a flight. We went to the toilet with a changing board and played the same song that we always play at home. I changed her diaper, washed her, etc., then put her sleeping bag on and gave her a bottle feed while she was sitting on my lap. The plane was already dark, which made a big difference. The first time flying, she slept in a cot the flight attendants attached to the wall in front of us. So, after the whole evening ritual we sang the same lullaby as we did at home and said 'night, night'. She fell asleep right away. No hassle, no hours of crying; Liv knew exactly what she had to do. I found it to be the ultimate proof that structure and regularity works well with our child. We were so happy and relieved.

Child-friendly accommodation

You might find it convenient to book a hotel, apartment, or campsite where you can do your own laundry. If you do this, you won't have to take tons of clothes, underwear, and baby clothes with you; after all, you already have to take so much stuff when you travel with kids. Your laundry will dry quickly if you're in a hot climate, and it saves you lots of work when you get home.

I always read the recommendations for the hotel or apartment we want to go to. While looking for an accommodation, I make sure to check the 'child friendly' box in the search field. Once I've found a hotel that appeals to me, I read the reviews religiously, because sometimes hotels claim to be child friendly but there's a noisy bar on the other side of the road, or the staff isn't child friendly at all. These are things you want to know up front. If you've been looking forward to your first family holiday, you don't want to be disappointed by annoying things that you could have avoided.

CHAPTER 15

Round Two?

A mother's love
Is whole
No matter how many
Times it is divided

On reflection, I realise that before I became a mom I wasn't very happy: I was insecure and very restless. I rushed from one thing to another and could barely stand to be alone. I even ended up suffering from burnout a few years before Liv was born. I needed to learn how to prioritize myself and how to love myself unconditionally. I think going through PPD taught me to finally be able to do that. As crazy as it might sound, I'm actually grateful I went through it all because it taught me so much about myself, about the kind of mother I want to be, and how to take better care of myself.

Before becoming a mom, self-care was never on the menu. I was forever using up my energy, my last resources in order to achieve my goals. It always had to *be* better; I always had to *do* better. It was insane. Instead of fuelling myself and loving myself for who I am, I aimed for the highest goals, which (of course) I would never achieve and then I would beat myself up about it. These days I see myself as an improved version of Tilda. I lowered the bar a lot for myself and I now know that good is good enough. I no longer aim for perfection, because I know it's not important. I love myself for who I am now, and I set some serious boundaries for myself. Because if I can't do it, who will? Or: No one else is going to do this, so I have to do this for myself.

When Livia was two and a half, something truly unexpected happened. I was sitting on the couch one night and suddenly felt this unstoppable longing to have another baby. I didn't know what was happening to me. Even though I had recovered from PPD by then, I had always assumed we wouldn't have another child. I felt so confused and at the same time so happy.

Tim came home from work and sat next to me on the couch. I said, 'I'm going to say something really crazy.' He looked at me warily. I said, 'I think I want another baby.' I looked at him shyly, a little scared about how he might react. He looked at me with a big smile on his face. 'I'm going to say something crazy as well…I think I want another one, too.' We beamed at each other, both of us touched by our feelings. I was so surprised by his reaction. I couldn't believe we both had this feeling out of the blue at the same time, because normally we're very different in our opinions and how we experience things. So it was wonderful!

We started talking about all the 'what ifs'. What if I get PPD again? What if I spiral back into that black sinkhole? What if I don't want to breastfeed again? What if I experience another traumatic birth? You name it, we talked about it. We chatted for hours and both agreed that we felt very strongly about protecting me from PPD. We decided I wasn't going to breastfeed again because the first time was such a disaster. The second thing was sleep. I don't do well on little sleep. Tim would take two weeks off to help me and do the night feeds so I could recover from the birth. We talked about what kind of delivery I wanted, and I felt I wanted a C-section, because of the previous birth trauma. We made a solid plan for how we would handle everything once I got pregnant again.

After a couple of months, we started trying. It had taken me almost two years to get pregnant with Livia, so I wasn't expecting to get pregnant fast. But miracles happen. I got pregnant on our second try. Watching that pregnancy test turn positive was incredible. I was so thrilled! I got Tim into the bathroom and we just stood there holding each other, hugging, kissing, and looking at that positive test result in our hands. Livia was going to be a big sister.

Dear moms, after reading this book you know a lot about the more difficult aspects of motherhood. Maybe you've read things you didn't (want to) know, and maybe you realized that much of what you're going through is common to other women, too. I want you to know that if you're not feeling well after giving birth to your first child, it doesn't mean it will go that way with your second baby. Everything could be fine, as it was with me. My experience was totally different the second time. I was feeling so much better mentally and it wasn't such a sh*t show as with the first time.

When I look back on the period after Livia was born, I just want to give the old me a hug and tell her it'll all be okay in the end. Although right now you might not be able to even imagine feeling happy ever again, *you will*. Giving yourself grace, giving yourself unconditional self-love is what you need when you go through postpartum depression. Don't beat yourself up because you're feeling a certain way. You're allowed to have all these feelings. Becoming a mother is fantastic, it's a revelation, it's everything. And, yes, it's also brutal sometimes. That keeps it balanced, doesn't it? Please be kind to yourself, because you're doing the best you can.

I want you to have faith in yourself, in your capabilities as a woman, as a mother, and as a human being. You are enough! Even if you don't feel like it. You're your baby's favourite person. You're your child's rock. You're the one he turns to when he's feeling blue. Start looking for evidence of why you *are* a good mother instead of why you're supposing you're not. Once you start digging for negativity, something will always come up. We're good that way. But is that helpful? No! So please try and focus on the good. That's all that matters.

ACKNOWLEDGEMENTS

First of all, I want to thank The Dreamwork Collective for believing in my book. Kira and her team, you guys are truly fantastic! Heike Schüssler, thank you for the beautiful cover and being open to my ideas.

Thalia, my wonderful, amazing, kind-hearted editor. You've made this book into what it was meant to be. You were my beacon in the night and I couldn't have done this without you. I am forever grateful. Thank you so much.

Thank you to all the moms out there who have been supporting and following me: I'm so blessed to have you in my corner.

To my family and all my friends, it's an amazing feeling to have you as my tribe, my coven, and my support. You've showed me that friends are family that you chose yourself. You were with me from the start and have supported me whenever I needed it. I love you all.

My dearest, sweetest Livia and Emmi, you are the lights in my life. Thank you for making me a mommy and for teaching me new lessons each day. Thanks to you two, I'm the person I have become. You're the reason I wrote this book and you make my world a beautiful place. I love you so incredibly much.

And last but most certainly not least, to my husband, Tim. You are my rock, my heart and soul, and the love of my life. I couldn't have done any of this if it wasn't for you. The love that I feel for you is endless and I'm so blessed to have you in my life. I love you to the moon and back.

NOTES

1. https://www.nimh.nih.gov/health/publications/
postpartum-depression-facts/index.shtml

2. https://www.psychologiemagazine.nl/artikel/
kwade-gedachten/

3. https://www.huffingtonpost.co.uk/entry/new-parents
-gender-disappointment_uk_58f8a3e6e4b091e58f38ba49

4. http://www.nu.nl/gezondheid/3856658/borstvoeding
-halveert-risico-postnatale-depressie.html

5. https://www.telegraph.co.uk/news/2017/08/29/exercise
-can-help-new-mothers-manage-postnatal-depression-study/

6. https://st-josef-apotheke.de/

7. https://www.emdr.com/what-is-emdr/

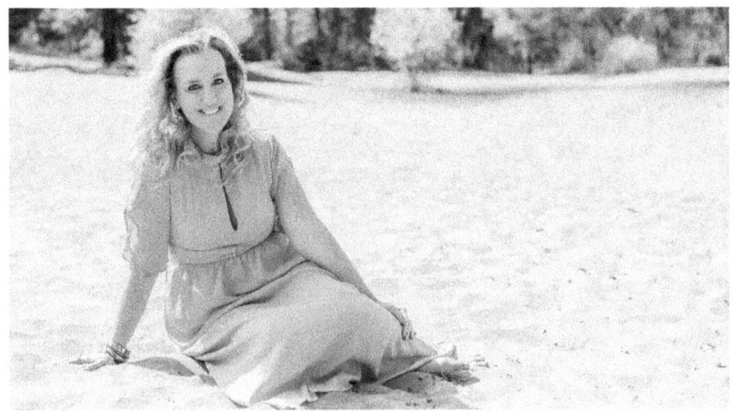

Tilda Timmers

Netherlands-based Tilda Timmers is a therapist specialising in postpartum depression. She works with parents who are not on cloud nine after giving birth, who might be feeling over-whelmed, ashamed, depressed, and anything in between. She helps give them their life back, introducing them to tools they need to feel more confident, happier and balanced in their new role as a parent.

Tilda writes from the heart having suffered from postpartum depression with her first child. Her dream is to help as many parents as she can to get through what might be their biggest challenge to date.

@thisispostpartum

www.ingramcontent.com/pod-product-compliance
Lightning Source LLC
Chambersburg PA
CBHW071606150726
48000CB00004B/1610